Lisa Lynch was a journalist and magazine editor. At the age of 28, while editing her second interiors title, Lisa discovered a lump in her breast – a lump that spawned not just cancer, but a blog (www.alrighttit.com), this book and a writing career.

Follow the blog at www.alrighttit.com

www.lisalynch.co.uk

THE
C-WORD

Just your average 28-year old... Friends,
Family, Facebook, Cancer

Lisa Lynch

arrow books

First published by Arrow Books in 2010
This edition published by Arrow Books, 2015

6 8 10 9 7 5

Arrow Books
Random House, 20 Vauxhall Bridge Road,
London SW1V 2SA

www.rbooks.co.uk

Addresses for companies within The Random House Group Limited can
be found at: www.randomhouse.co.uk

The Random House Group Limited Reg. No. 954009

A CIP catalogue record for this book
is available from the British Library

ISBN 9781784750473

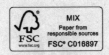

Typeset by SX Composing DTP, Rayleigh, Essex
Printed and bound by CPI Group (UK) Ltd, Croydon, CR0 4YY

For Cyril and Jean

A note from Pete

I first met Lisa at work, and I recall asking her what she did. 'I'm a sub editor,' she said enthusiastically. I probed her a little on what this involved and I came away enlightened. It was, aside from family, music and writing, her number one passion. Whilst one person's nirvana might be a cocktail on a secluded Caribbean beach, Lisa's was implementing a house style for the magazine she worked on and making bad copy good (don't get me wrong, she loved a good holiday too, like).

We had been happily married for a year when the C bomb was dropped into our world and Lisa turned to one of her first loves. She wrote. When she first picked up her MacBook and started writing what became her blog and later this book, she'd often turn to me and say, 'Love, will you check this before I post it?' I would (nervously) check it and then hand it back to her with a knowing smile: there was never anything to spot – Lisa Lynch copy was always *thoroughly* checked.

You can imagine, then, what my initial reaction was when invited to write this introduction. Must-ask-Lisa-what-to-do. It's a course of action that has served me very well over the years in more matters than I'd dare to admit and it's one that I still stick to.

By now, you'll know why I was invited to write this, and it never gets any easier to say: Lisa died very peacefully on March 11, 2013. Since then, for me anyway, the world has seemed a lot less interesting. I posted on her blog during the days following her death that her 'light would never go out' and that I think is what sustains me and, I know, her family.

You see, the thing is, she prepared us for this and forever told us to carry on; to do the things we always did; to squeeze everything we can out of life. That is precisely what we are doing because that's what she did. I suggest you do the same, but before you do, please please read her story because it will inspire you along the way.

Peter
August, 2014

Contents

Introduction

On my lengthy 'Things To Do Before I'm Thirty' list (see Northern Lights, get pregnant, write book, lose stone, own Christian Louboutins), I hadn't factored in beating breast cancer. But them's the breaks.

The ball-ache was less about having to add such a hefty task to my list than it was about the sheer bloody inconvenience of it taking precious time out of my late twenties. I had lots of very serious business to attend to, thank you very much, like shopping sprees and Wonderbra-wearing and romantic weekends away and getting drunk over dinner with mates (not that that'd help on the losing-a-stone front, mind). But while I had to concede that The Bullshit (as I've come to refer to it) would have to come first for a while, I was determined to get the good times back, and not allow it to take away anything more than my hair. (And let's be honest, that was pissing on my chips quite enough.)

I've always worked on the assumption that, whatever it is, it's better to know about it. (The truth may hurt, but it's always preferable to know when your skirt is tucked into your knickers, right?) Nor have I ever been one for keeping my mouth shut. So I started a blog, *Alright Tit*, on which I kept a journal of my cancer experience. And writing while fighting is a strategy that's worked – not only have my friends and family been kept informed on all the stuff they'd never hear from Kylie (or Brave Kylie, to give her her full name), but it's also been a cathartic method of keeping me out of the therapist's chair (for the most part).

I'm not pretending to be the only twenty-something in the world who's had a breast cancer diagnosis. I'm just probably the one with the biggest gob. But everyone needs a strategy, and mine has been to write my way through The Bullshit (and come out the other side walking taller in a fabulous pair of Louboutins).

*

Carrie Bradshaw fell in Dior, I fell in Debenhams. It was May 2008, and it was spectacular. Uncomfortable heels + slippy floor + head turned by a cocktail dress = *thwack*. Arms stretched overhead, teeth cracking on floor tiles, chest and knees breaking the fall, legs flailing about like a mid-tantrum toddler. It was theatrical, exaggerated, a perfect 6.0. And it was Significant Moment #1 in discovering that I had grade-three breast cancer.

Significant Moment #2 came a month later, when my husband and I were play-fighting. On the outside, we're a professional London-based couple with mortgage protection, a cafetiere and one eye on our Air Miles. Behind closed doors, we draw on one another's foreheads, have noisy Beatles-album sing-offs and tickle each other until we can't breathe for laughing. Attempting to fight back while slowly losing each of my nerve endings and trying to hang

2

onto a full bladder, I thought I'd buy myself some time by adding 'and remember I'm still in pain from my fall' to the 'I'm a girl, go easy on me' card I'd already played. But when you're married to The Most Competitive Man In The World, such pathetic excuses mean nothing, and he went in for the kill by holding my arms behind my back and reaching for my Debenhams-bruised left boob. When P called time on our scrap because the playful boob-grab had hurt me more than it ought to, and he'd copped a feel of more than his usual handful, I knew something was wrong. (P never gives up first.) And that was precisely the moment at which the fun stopped, and my cancer journey began.

Actually, that's an odd choice of words, since I loathe the term 'journey' when applied to cancer. Journey implies a pleasant trip to the seaside, a magical mystery tour or an epiphany during some life-changing experience. Cancer isn't a journey. Cancer is a nuclear bomb dropped in the centre of your lovely world – in this case with sod all warning. There's nothing liberating or celebratory or enlightening about it.

Being diagnosed with cancer is like being told you've got twenty minutes to revise for an A level in a language you've never learned. (*Parlez-vous chemo?*) You walk into your appointment assuming your cramming days are behind you, and come out blinded by need-to-know, baffling terminology that's as unfamiliar as a snowman to a Fijian. The literature is all so delicately written; packed with non-committal information ('you might find . . .', 'there's a possibility that . . .', 'you may discover . . . ', 'if you feel . . .'), and a sugary, hey-it's-really-not-so-bad attitude, like a flimsy net curtain attempting to disguise a bloody great elephant.

I don't want to be told that losing my hair will give me

3

extra time in bed in the morning where I'd otherwise have been blow-drying, or that buying a range of wigs will give me the chance to try out different personalities in the bedroom (both of which I read in an 'uplifting compilation of quotes' from breast cancer survivors). Nor do I want to give anyone else that impression. It's irresponsible and, frankly, it's complete crap – even before I'd experienced any of the things the contributors were talking about, I knew that wasn't how it was going to be. I'd have given up all the lie-ins in the world to keep my lovely locks. And not only do chemo drugs tend to starve you of a sex life, but breast cancer treatment hardly does wonders for your body image either. (I don't recall ever seeing a twenty-something lass with a bald head and missing boob on *FHM*'s '100 Sexiest Women' list.)

So stuff the clichéd, just-not-fucking-funny cancer quips ('think of all the money/time/effort you'll save on mascara/your hair/shaving your legs'), the saccharine, truth-masking 'information' sheets and the earnest, life-improving self-help books. It's time someone told it how it *really* is.

And that's precisely what I've done.

CHAPTER 1

An apology

June 2008

From a lack of decent conversation and a tendency to curiosity, my first (unsuitable) boyfriend and I fell into a routine of rarely speaking and instead used each other for experimentation. It didn't always feel good and wasn't always done right, but we were fifteen and fed up and keen to impress our mates. One over-enthusiastic afternoon in an otherwise empty house, I somehow ended up with a hurt right nipple. How? God knows. But the subsequent few weeks were experimentation-free, while the boob-scab healed and my unsuitable boyfriend found someone else to experiment with.

Thirteen years on, and I still silently blame this episode for my right boob being my least favourite. Not by a long chalk, mind – I've always been happy with my lot boobs-wise, and reckon that the few people who've seen them have been bloody lucky to do so – but we all play favourites, right? (Or left?)

And so today, I'd like to make an apology to my right breast. First off, for calling it a 'breast' just then. 'Breast' is just one of those words that I inexplicably hate, hence the inverted commas.

But mostly, I'd like to apologise to my right boob (ah, infinitely better) for always preferring the left, when that's the one that's gone and got cancer.

Is it too late to switch sides?

*

'Another G&T, Lis?'

Me and my mates had met up for a swift half (translation: three hours' worth of booze on an empty stomach) outside our favourite London pub. It was that glorious, once-a-year evening when the weather was finally good enough to swap leggings and boots for bare legs and open-toed wedges, and I was feeling good. I was wearing my first summer dress of the season, had covered my pins in suspiciously gravy-like fake tan and had just styled my newly grown-out fringe into the kind of sweeping side parting that makes you feel like Jessica Rabbit (but actually makes you look like you've only got one eye).

'Better not,' I answered to a jury of baffled looks. 'Seriously. I'm at the doctors in the morning. I've got a cyst that's giving me gyp in my tit, here.' For some reason I pointed to the offending boob; one too many G&Ts insisting that I give my friends a biology lesson. Nobody seemed the least bit concerned. I wasn't either. Because a lump in your tit at my age is *obviously* a cyst, right? And anyway, I was much more perturbed that my early appointment was putting paid to me pushing on till last orders. 'Let's catch up when I'm back from my hols, eh? When I've got a *real* tan to show off,' I said, kicking out a streaky orange leg and slinging my bag over my shoulder while zigzagging my way to the nearest available taxi.

The concern didn't even stretch to my GP. 'Yep, I'm sure

6

it's a cyst,' she said. 'It'll have disappeared by the time you're back from your holiday.'

P and I had spent months planning our trip: first to LA to visit Ant, one of my best mates, and then on to Mexico for some serious Corona-drinking, sun-worshipping, nacho-scoffing relaxation. Secretly, we both assumed it would also be where we struck pregnancy gold. (Following two miscarriages in six months, baby-making was fast becoming an obsessive pursuit.) So neither of us was prepared to let a pesky, pain-in-the-arse (nay, boob) cyst ruin our sun-filled shagging schedule.

But one week of uncomfortable bikini-wearing and batting P's hand away from my left boob later, and the lump had begun to worry me. It was hardening, painful to the touch and, frankly, ruining the line of my spaghetti-strap summer dresses. I mentioned it to Ant.

'Can you move it about?' she asked as we ate our fro-yo on Venice Boardwalk. I slipped my hand beneath my top and poked the lump, figuring that with Muscle Beach directly opposite, nobody would notice a pale Brit fondling her left tit.

'Um, yeah, I guess so,' I said, wondering whether too much prodding might cause the lump to explode like a shampoo bottle at high altitude.

'Then it'll be a cyst,' she assured me. 'Have it checked out again when you get back and I bet they can even remove it there and then.'

And so I did, albeit not immediately. For while we were in Mexico, we received the news I'd been dreading ever since my beloved Nan died the year before: Grandad had joined her. It's particularly strange getting that kind of call on a balcony overlooking the ocean in the blistering morning sun. Your folks explain what's happened, then eventually run out of stuff to say, forcing normal conversation with 'are you having a nice time?' and 'what's the weather like?', neither of which you know how to answer. I wanted to come home immediately, but nobody was having it. There were only a few days left until we were heading back anyway and, as this was something we'd all been expecting for months, there was nothing in particular I could have done. And so I sobbed in the sunshine until I got back on home soil, where I sobbed in the drizzle instead. With a funeral to arrange and attend, and a thousand brilliant stories of Grandad's days as Derbyshire's grumpiest cricket umpire (The Grumpire) to tell, the cyst would have to wait. Not that I was worrying about it any longer anyway. If bad luck had been on the way, losing Grandad was surely it.

A week after his funeral, I finally got around to getting my lump looked at once more. I headed back to see my GP, forcefully suggesting that if it wasn't a cyst, it must instead be the early signs of pregnancy. (Having twice been knocked up, I knew that the hormones would shoot straight to my bust.) 'You might be right,' she said, rubbing her fit-to-burst baby bump. 'But I'm going to send you for a needle biopsy anyway, just in case.'

Everything froze. Either I'd suddenly found myself in an episode of *Heroes*, with Hiro Nakamura-style powers of time-stopping, or my GP has just used the word 'biopsy'.

'Sorry, um . . . biopsy?' I stuttered, still sitting bra-less and bolt-upright on the bed. She gestured to me to get dressed, assuring me that it was nothing to lose sleep about, given my age (twenty-eight) and zero family history of breast cancer. Even the eight-week NHS wait for the needle biopsy (standard for 'low-risk' cases) didn't concern her. But, adding mention of the word 'biopsy' to my tendency to procrastinate my way to insomnia after as little as a late-night episode of *24*, an eight-week wait seemed like a millennia, and I asked for a referral to a private specialist. Eight weeks shrank to forty-eight hours.

P had come with me to my second GP appointment – perhaps more for an early finish from work than out of any serious concern – and we took our chance to enjoy the late-afternoon sun as London's commuters made their way home. Supping our lager shandies on a bench outside our local pub, we faked nonchalance as best we could, making light of the biopsy that weekend. Once a year, P has to work Saturdays and this, of course, was it. 'No bother,' I said, 'It'll just be a quick in-and-out with a needle. They can't shed any light on it then anyway.'

I called my folks when P went in for another pint. 'So she's sending me for a needle biopsy on Saturday,' I recounted breezily, to uncharacteristic silence.

'Right,' said Mum, eventually. 'Um, okay. I see. Right. How are you getting there?'

'Well, I've got the car because P's at work so I'll just drive myself round,' I said, sensing the worry in her voice but thinking little of it, given that Mum has a tendency to fret in much the same way if I mention that I'm crossing the road, getting on the night bus or meeting a friend for a drink.

Dad was in the background, butting in. 'Tell her we'll come down tomorrow night. Tell her we can be there in the morning if she needs us.' Mum reiterated his words.

'No, it's fine,' I insisted. 'Stop worrying.'

I told P how Mum had sounded. 'Your mum's a worrier by nature,' he said. 'Look at you; you're fine. Everything's going to be fine.'

As it happened, that Saturday was far from fine, but not necessarily because of the biopsy. The morning had begun

9

with one of the only two rows P and I ever have (the other being our regular Paul v John Battle of The Beatles): he'd rolled in narnared at 3 a.m. – which wouldn't have been a problem had he not told me he'd be home by 11.30 and dropped his BlackBerry in a urinal – and I'd started an already twitchy day by giving him the hairdryer treatment for leaving me fretting like a nervy mother at midnight on her teenage son's first night out on the town. He headed out to work, a furious flea ringing in his ear, and I drove to the hospital, more than a little pissed off.

In the tiny consultation room, I was met with the now-standard reassuring words – again citing my age and lack of family history – as the smartly dressed consultant sunk a needle into my boob. He wrote his number on a business card. 'I'm sure I can get the results by as early as Tuesday,' he told me. 'Give my secretary a call and she'll squeeze you in that afternoon.' And, jolt as it was that I'd have answers so soon, I figured it was better than two months' worth of crankiness and nail-biting.

As I drove home, I thought about the following week's unusually busy schedule at the branded content agency in which I was an editor – client meeting all day on Monday, press deadline on Tuesday – and for once found myself grateful to have so much to occupy my time. A noise distracted me from my thought. Clack-clack-clack. 'What the . . .?' I said, as I noticed the driver behind me gesturing wildly, making downward-pointing motions with his index finger. 'What's your problem, dude?' I snapped into my rear-view mirror, speeding up a bit down the hill that leads to my street.

The noise continued. Clack-clack-clack. I made it back to the flat and, climbing out of the car as I jerked the handbrake, spotted the flat tyre. 'Bollocks,' I spat, a little too loudly for my quiet suburban street, and headed into the flat to ditch my bag and call P. As his phone rang, I went back out to the car to survey the damage, angrily slamming the front door behind me. Another expletive echoed around my neighbourhood. 'Tiiits!' My keys were still in my handbag. The kid next door stuck his head over the fence and grinned, mischievously impressed by my swearing. I left a few more on P's answerphone, and couldn't help but wonder if this was the universe's wicked way of forecasting a shitstorm.

Each busy at work over the following couple of days, P and I did our best to keep ourselves occupied at home, too, avoiding talking about the obvious by going out for dinner on the Monday night with Mum, who was staying over prior to a conference in London. Whenever conversation turned to the following day, the three of us would robotically recite the consultant's reassurances like some sort of panic-avoiding mantra.

'So I'm going to have to shoot off a bit early tomorrow,' I'd told my boss earlier that day. 'I had a biopsy on a lump in my boob at the weekend and I'm getting the results.'

She looked up from the sink as we washed our hands in the toilets of our client's office. 'But it won't be anything to worry about, surely?'

I scrunched up my face and gave a little shake of the head. 'Probably a cyst,' I said. 'I'll be back in to check proofs on Wednesday morning.'

I wasn't.

'We're running a bit behind, but we'll do your mammogram as soon as the room's free,' said the nurse, crouching in front of us and resting her hand on my knee.

'She just touched my leg,' I whispered to P. 'I've never met her. What's all that about?'

Even the waiting room was confusing to me. I didn't even realise I was scheduled for a mammogram. P brushed off my suspicion. 'She's probably just a touchy-feely person; some nurses are like that,' he said unconvincingly, getting back to his BlackBerry while still gripping my left hand.

An hour passed. People who came in long after us were being seen almost immediately. I avoided asking the receptionist what was going on and instead opted for tutting loudly and craning my neck to see how often the door to the mammogram room was opening. Eventually, another nurse appeared from that end of the corridor. She handed me a gown and led me through the door, all the while gushing with compliments about my scuffed, red shoes. 'They're take-you-anywhere shoes, those,' she said, as I stood before the six-foot-high machine and she adjusted a flat, metal plate for me to rest my boob on.

'I guess so,' I said, more concerned about the second plate closing down above my bust.

'It's going to squeeze a bit, but it's only for a few seconds,' she explained as I sucked in sharp intakes of breath to stop myself from crying at the sight – and pain – of my tit being flattened like a piece of Play-Doh. 'I could do with some shoes like that,' she continued. 'The kind that'll take you to work and then the pub afterwards and not leave you with blisters. And red's such a versatile colour.' The machine whirred back to its resting position.

'Something's up here,' I thought. 'Nobody gets that excited about £12 cork wedges.' And suddenly the other nurse's knee-touch made sense. I was being primed for a cancer diagnosis.

Pulling my sequined star-motif T-shirt back on, the nurse

led P and me into my specialist's room, still impossibly chirpy and complimentary and high-pitched. There was a scan of my boobs on a wall-hung light box. I was amazed at how quickly it had got there; it reminded me of the time I broke my wrist at Rollerworld as a kid, and how exciting I found it at the hospital, looking at my X-rays, being put in plaster and pinning an 'I've been to casualty' badge to my sling. But, from the sombre look on the faces of my specialist and the nurse beside him, P and I could tell that my days of exciting hospital appointments had come to a whiplash-inducing halt.

From behind his imposing desk, my specialist pointed to a cloudy area on the scan, saying sentences I can't recall that could only point to one conclusion. I heard the words 'breast cancer'. The rest was white noise.

Talk about post-holiday blues. My tan has never faded so fast.

CHAPTER 2

Reality bites

'It's *probably* just a cyst. '

'I'm *sure* it will be completely benign. '

'*If* it turns out the cancer is invasive.'

'*In case* you require chemotherapy.'

'In the *unlikely event* that the CT scan shows cancer in other organs . . .'

Yadda yadda yadda. Will someone give me a straight answer, for fuck's sake?

Forgive my bleak outlook, but right now I'm struggling to hunt down the humour that fools everyone else into thinking I'm handling all this. Today, I'm not handling anything. All I can see at the moment is the fact that cancer kills. And before you start, don't go telling me that time is on my side, that breast cancer is really curable these days, that I'm a fighter . . . I'm well aware of all those things, thank you very much. And I also know that if you were in my patent pumps, you'd be looking at the bleakest outcome too.

*

'I don't understand what they told me,' I said to P as we

walked from the hospital to the car park. 'I can't take it in.'
I was on autopilot. P too. God knows how he managed to
drive us home.

'They told us the news,' he said. (At this early stage, none
of us could bring ourselves to say the word 'cancer', which
is how its replacement, 'The Bullshit', came about – the He
Who Must Not Be Named to cancer's Voldemort.) 'And then
they said that they'd need to determine whether it's
invasive or non-invasive. Non-invasive is better – you
might get away without chemotherapy then – but if it's
invasive, you're going to need chemotherapy and radiotherapy as soon as your mastectomy is out of the way.' I
couldn't get my head around the multi-syllable medical
vocab I was suddenly having to learn.

'And that's really necessary, is it, the mastectomy?' I spat,
as though it were P who'd decided that it must be done.

'It is, babe,' he said, ignoring my barbed tone. 'They'll
give you the date for that when we go back in on Friday for
the results of your core biopsy.'

The core biopsy was a bitch. Before having it, but right
after getting 'the news', I'd been led out of the room by the
professor and nurse who broke it to me and handed a cup
of tea. I'd say that both P and I were in tears, but in fact we
were doing that kind of crying that comes without tears.
Startled crying. Confused crying. Frozen-to-your-core,
terrified crying. The kind of crying that sends your body
into such paralysing, world-stopping shock that your tear
ducts can't function, so you just sniff and wail and tremble,
like an actor who can't produce the good stuff on cue.

P stared at his BlackBerry. 'Shit,' he said, looking up at me
with yet another level of terror in his eyes. 'Your mum and
dad. I've missed a ton of calls.' Fuck. Mum and Dad. How
was I going to tell them? As we sat in the hospital, Mum

would have been on the train back from a day-long London conference to my hometown of Derby, where Dad would soon be driving to the local station to pick her up. We'd been in the hospital for almost four hours. They'd both been calling the entire time. And since I always – *always* – make time to speak to my folks every day, whether from airport runways, drunken karaoke sessions or mud-soaked Glastonbury fields, the fact that they'd not been able to get hold of me could only mean one thing.

'We can't call Mum while she's on the train,' I said to P, subtly suggesting with a 'we' that it wasn't a given that I would be making the call. 'We'll have to speak to Dad.' And so we did. No – P did.

Another nurse appeared to take me for my core biopsy, and P nodded as I was led away. 'I'll do it now,' he said, in a show of selfless courage that was to become typical of his behaviour throughout The Bullshit. I don't know what was said in that phone call. I don't *ever* want to know what was said in that phone call.

Feeling helplessly guilty that my stupid, stupid body was soon to break the hearts of my dad, mum and brilliant kid brother Jamie, just as it had my husband before them, I headed into the small, dark room, sat on the bed and stripped to the waist, still snivelling and shaking and stupefied. The nurse explained how the core biopsy was going to work, but of course I wasn't listening, and so it came as an excruciating shock when what can only be described as an apple corer shot into my bust, pulling with it a sample of the tumour that was threatening to ruin my life, and leaving me bruised and swollen. All the while I stared, moist-eyed, at a watercolour painting on the opposite wall. To this day, I loathe watercolours.

'Did you call him?' I asked P as I walked back into the

waiting room, though I could tell from his grey pallor that he had. I retched at the thought of P's words bringing my dad – my brilliant Dad; the one person in the world I most want to be like – such woe with the news that no parent can prepare themselves for. 'You need to call him,' P replied solemnly as we walked out of the clinic, bidding the professor and his nurse a purposeful goodbye as we left. (A cancer diagnosis, I've discovered, tends to enhance Britishness – pleasantries, talk of the weather, cups of tea . . . as though in a crisis, politeness is all we have left.)

It's funny what your brain forgets. More than 'everything's going to be okay', I can't remember what I told my dad on the phone as P and I drove home from the hospital. Nor can I remember what I told Mum when I later spoke to her. Nor the reactions of my closest friends, who were on the receiving end of the same kind of phone call. Not even the words of my boss, who I called at home that night.

I recently asked my family what they remember of that day, expecting to hear meticulous, blow-by-blow stories of exactly what was said, what the weather was like and what song was on the radio. But not even they can recount any details. Mum remembers little more than 'a feeling of absolute terror'. Dad remembers his head being 'scrambled' and trying to hold it together while talking to P, but breaking down as soon as he ended the call. Jamie assumed that Mum must have been wrong when she said 'it's cancer', but abruptly thought 'fuck me, it's real' when he saw Dad in tears two steps behind. And P? Well, P was with me. And short of disbelief, confusion and a sudden inability to swallow, his recollection is as sketchy as mine.

It's by no means a perfect account of those bleak few hours – certainly not enough for a *Crimewatch* reconstruction, say, or a *Match of the Day* highlights package –

but those snatched film stills, those tiny moments in time, are what remain on the editing-room floor. It's as though our minds have wiped it all like a hard drive we'd hoped to protect; as though what was stored is of no use to us; as though we're better off without it. And I'm grateful. I *want* to be protected from that stuff, from those painful moments that punctuated the beginning of The Bullshit. The phone calls, the conversations, the moment I first saw my parents after they'd thrown what they could into a case, dropping off keys and terrible news with Jamie, before heading down to London as quickly as the speed cameras of the M40 would allow them.

Something neither my brain – nor my hard drive – has wiped, however, was the embarrassingly cop-out, multi-recipient email I sent to the friends I hadn't told in a phone call.

Subject: Well here I am to stuff up your Wednesday morning.

Hi everyone

First off, please forgive the group mailer. I won't beat about the bush here as this is a difficult enough email to send, so here's the thing: I have breast cancer. We're hoping it's only early stages and while it's very unusual to get it at my age, I'm told that's actually going to help me in getting over it. I had a core biopsy yesterday which will determine whether the cancer is invasive or non-invasive (we're gunning for the latter), and that in turn will determine my course of treatment. Either way, after Friday they'll get straight round to it treatment-wise and it'll be easier all round (she says, naively) because we can be practical about it all, rather than emotional (and to be honest, I can't be dealing with the emotional side of

it). So that's my news. Sorry to those of you who I'm
suddenly back in touch with thanks to this bullshit, and
I promise I'll keep you all posted as much as I can. Now
for fuck's sake, someone tell an inappropriate joke or
something.
Lis xxx

I can't help but shake my head and snigger patronisingly at
that email. The ill-prepared, misinformed, simplified,
cancer's-messing-with-the-wrong-girl tone makes me
cringe. I was stupidly ignorant. But what did I know? At that
moment, I'd hoped my cancer was early stages, non-
invasive and treatable with little more than a mastectomy.
My follow-up appointment that Friday revealed a different
story.

With Mum and Dad staying at the flat, we somehow filled
the two days before my appointment with the strangest of
time-occupying tasks: sizing up mini TVs in Dixons so
they'd have something to watch in the box room that was
to become their second home; choosing a mattress topper
in Ikea to make the sofabed more comfortable; pyjama-
buying in Marks & Spencer because Mum insisted my
mismatched rock t-shirt and shorts combos weren't
suitable for a five-day stay in hospital. It's very typical of my
family, this kind of behaviour – met with a crisis, we
immediately turn to the practicalities. We'd say it's a
Midlands thing, but maybe it's typical of most families? Yes,
there's been a cancer diagnosis, but there's still laundry to
do, mugs to wash, weeds to pull up and *Coronation Street*
to watch. These simple, seemingly inane, minute-passers
are what I and my family do best. (Run out of hot water,
forget the matchday parking ticket, or churn up the lawn
with an enthusiastic summertime kickabout, however, and

it's meltdown time.) It was our way of making things better, of striving for an indifference to the pain. We couldn't change the fact that I had cancer, but we could ensure that we had everything in place to make this as smooth a ride as possible, whether it be new pillows or extra teabags or limescale remover for the shower screen.

The problem with that tactic, however, is that you can fill up your days with pointless activities as much as you like, but the emotion's going to have to come out at some point, and so the rest of those sombre, surreal forty-eight hours was filled with the kind of agonising and wretched heart-break that makes you unable to speak or eat or stop yourself from crying noisily in the middle of a busy M&S café. Then sadness turns to anger. Mum shouted at a changing room attendant for not allowing us both into the same cubicle. I erupted into a tantrum when the spotty pyjamas she'd brought me to try on made me 'look like an ill person'. Dad got frustrated with the instruction manuals of the various gadgets he'd bought to keep me occupied in hospital. All we each longed for was something – *anything* – to blame, but shop staff, pyjamas and iPod speakers fell disappointingly short of the mark, and rage morphed back into frustrated, confused despair.

Why we thought shopping was a good idea, I'll never know. Even at the best of times, we're not a family who shops well together. For us, the therapy in 'retail therapy' is about as exciting a prospect as the therapy in 'chemotherapy'. Mum is famously short-tempered. Dad is famously uninterested. And I'm famously impatient with their short temper and disinterest. But I guess that in such an otherwise bewildering time, shopping represented something normal. And all we each wanted more than anything else was to enforce some normality on the

20

situation, even though everything happening around us was anything but.

We'd get back to the flat after our shopping missions and I'd immediately disappear under my duvet fully clothed, lasting little more than twenty minutes before realising that, actually, I needed company, whether or not I made the most of it. Not that we ever made the most of each other's company when we weren't out on pointless shopping trips. We rarely did more than sit and stare at each other – me on the sofa, Dad in the armchair, Mum on the ottoman in the bay window – with baffled tears running down our cheeks until P came home from work, and he joined in too.

But even being surrounded by my favourite people in the world felt hopelessly lonely, because nobody knew what it was like to be stuck in my tortured mind and my useless body – nor was I keen to tell them. I needed an escape. Some people confide in a therapist, but I didn't have one. Some people go to confession, but I'd never been to church. Some people talk to their cats, but I wasn't an animal person. If this had been anything other than cancer – a problem with work, say, or a relationship issue – I'd have instinctively spoken to my family and friends about it. But not only was I completely SICK of talking about cancer after mere days of it being in my stratosphere, but its arrival had given each of my confidantes enough of a shock already, and adding my bleak thoughts to that horrible reality wouldn't have made them or me feel any better. And so my mind was close to capacity with unspoken thoughts and fears and questions and worries and emotions and frustrations, which I had no idea how or where to download.

Until Thursday afternoon, when an email I was writing somehow turned into more of a narrative, and it became clear that I'd turned to my Mac for comfort. (It would never have happened on a PC.) And forgive me for offering such a wanky explanation, but writing about the frustrating, life-altering, sheer bloody pain-in-the-arse place in which I found myself seemed the natural thing to do. I wasn't consciously keeping a diary; I wasn't even consciously starting a blog – but with more thoughts swimming around my head than I could hold on to, I needed to put them somewhere, and my keyboard offered an easy solution.

I momentarily flattered myself that I could become the Carrie Bradshaw of breast cancer – all long mousy hair, cross-legged on a bed, dreaming of shoes and baring all to a MacBook. But then reality called, and I looked up to find myself not in a couture-filled Upper East Side apartment, but a bargain-crammed flat in Wandsworth. And as much as I might have convinced myself that White Company pyjama bottoms are the height of sophistication, I doubt they could make quite the same style statement as a pink tutu.

And so I passed the time until the following Friday's consultation by writing my cancer-column. 'Whatever it is,' I assured everyone before the appointment, 'it's better to know about it. Then we can get back to being practical instead of working ourselves up by guessing.'

P and I introduced my folks to the professor and nurse who we'd seen the previous Tuesday.

'Oh, it *is* good that you've got your parents around you,' said the nurse as she shook my dad's hand. 'Long may it continue,' she added enigmatically, as my mum clocked her meaning. 'I'm sorry to keep you waiting, Lisa,' she said, turning to me, 'but Prof wants to see the easy ones first; he'd like to spend a bit more time with you.'

I turned to P, then to my folks, as the nurse walked away. Dad later told me that the look on my face will haunt him for the rest of his life. 'Well, that's it, then,' I grunted, defeated. 'She's preparing me for the worst.' Nobody disagreed. We all knew that I was about to hear the word 'invasive'.

That wasn't all P and I heard. Back in his office, the professor pointed with his rollerball to a diagram of a breast that reminded me of a GCSE Biology paper. He explained that my five-centimetre – *five centimetre!* – tumour wasn't just invasive, that it was not, in fact, early stages at all, but likely to be grade two or three, depending on whether he discovered a spread to my lymph nodes during my mastectomy.

'How many grades are there?' I asked, a cancer novice desperate to learn more.

'Four,' said the nurse.

'Shit,' I exhaled, quickly apologising for the expletive I'd let slip. I pulled my chair forward and rested both forearms on the professor's desk, my hands flat out on the dark oak, meaning business. 'What I can't understand,' I asserted, oddly cold and businesslike, 'is how I didn't find this sooner. How neither of us found this sooner,' I continued, gesturing to P. 'I mean, it's five centimetres!'

The professor drew more shapes on the breast diagram to demonstrate how the tumour had been growing immediately beneath my nipple, and had only begun to push out to the side – the side where P and I discovered it – as it had grown.

Mum couldn't hide her disbelief either. 'How didn't anybody pick this up?' she shrieked at the nurse, accusatorily. 'How can it be a cyst one moment and a huge, invasive tumour the next?' I was mortified.

'Let me fetch you all some tea and I'll answer your

questions,' said the nurse. It was clearly not the first time she'd been in such a situation.

'I just think it's *appalling* that nobody picked this up!' Mum yelled, getting louder and redder with every word. Dad was in pieces, clearly having the same angry thoughts but physically unable to verbalise them due to the wails that were choking him. P's head was held in his quivering hands as he stared at the patch of carpet that was soaking up his grief-stricken tears. And all of this was my doing. It was my body, my breast, my cancer that had sent my mum insanely livid, my dad deranged with distress and my husband into funereal melancholy. They were reacting as though I'd died, and yet there I sat, party to this tragic scene. I looked from Dad to Mum to P from Dad to P, to Mum. This was all too much. I was suffocating. I couldn't handle it.

'That's IT!' I screamed, propelling myself out of my plastic chair and kicking it back with my heel in one furious motion. 'I can't do this. I. CANT. DO. THIS!' They almost looked as surprised to see me there as they were at the sound of my outcry and the sight of me towering above them all, my bellowing words adding imposing inches to my 5 foot 7 frame. 'You have GOT to stop it. The lot of you! I know how hard this is – it's fucking IMPOSSIBLE – but I CANNOT HANDLE seeing you all like this.' (I figured now was as good a time as any to start saying 'fuck' in front of my parents.) 'I just CAN'T DEAL with this kind of emotion. So you can carry on being like you are and I'll deal with all of this on my own, or you can pack it in and do it with me. Because I CAN do this on my own, you know,' I continued haughtily, in what I knew even then was a massive fib. 'I can do it on my own and get through it all just fine, thank you, but what I CAN'T do is handle your emotion as well as my own, okay? OKAY? So what's it going to be?'

The nurse chose this moment to walk back into the room with tea and tissues. She looked pretty shell-shocked herself. Either she'd heard what was going on in there – hell, I'm sure most of Central London heard what was going on in there – or she was completely thrown by the stupefied silence that had descended on the room, thanks to my unexpected kick-ass outburst.

'Would you like me to explain everything again?' she asked my folks, who nodded calmly in agreement like two toddlers on the naughty step. This was for their benefit more than mine, although the nurse purposefully turned to me during the part about chemotherapy; the part that finished '. . . and you *will* lose your hair'.

I looked at Mum, crestfallen. She knew what I was thinking.

'I won't be able to go to Jamie's wedding,' I said. Jamie and Leanne's big day was four months away – slap-bang in the middle of my likely chemotherapy schedule.

'Of course you will,' said the nurse. 'You'll be able to wear a lovely long wig or a pretty headscarf and you'll look amazing.'

I ignored her assurances. I couldn't possibly turn up to such an important occasion in a wig. Wigs are for fancy dress, not weddings. And a headscarf? Don't be so bloody ridiculous. Who did she think I was, a fortune-teller? As she continued her recap of my diagnosis, my mind took a mental snapshot of the four of us beside the beautiful bride and the proud groom – Mum, Dad and P in their finery and then, standing awkwardly beside them, a balding, bloated George Dawes lookalike in a cocktail dress, ruining the photographs of my brother's happiest day for ever more.

CHAPTER 3

Let me get this off my chest

People keep telling me that I needn't keep 'being brave' and that I 'don't have to feel positive all the time' (get 'brave' and 'positive' on my Most Hated list IMMEDIATELY). They say that whenever I want to let it all out or get really angry or have a good cry, I can talk to them. And it's good of them to say so.

But let me say this for the record: I am not consciously *being* anything. I will never *want* to have a good cry or rant or whinge. Those things happen spontaneously: trying on pyjamas in Marks & Spencer, watering the garden, stirring my tea, blowing out a candle before I go to bed. At the moment, *every* reaction is spontaneous (hence a poor teenage shop assistant getting both barrels in Dixons recently).

In fact, this is the first fucking time in my whole life when I've stopped giving a shit about how I'm being, the way I'm acting or how I'm coming across to other people. Again: I am not trying to *be* anything, I'm just getting on with it.

None of these words, today or any other day, are for your benefit. I'm not 'being brave' to make you feel better. Repeat: I. Am. Not. Being. Brave. You needn't be concerned about how I'm coping. There is no 'how' here. I'm just coping. There's no good or bad way to do it. You'd cope too.

26

'Let's get something to eat before we go home,' I said to P and my folks as we left the hospital, still the reluctant flag-waving leader on our guided tour of cancer. After my chair-kicking outburst, they knew better than to suggest otherwise, and followed me in dazed single-file to the nearest restaurant, like unsteady newborn ducks being led to water by their plucky mother. We each pulled up a stool in The World's Worst Tapas Restaurant, throwing our bags and a rainforest's worth of breast cancer information leaflets onto the table. I hoped their presence would go some way to explaining our stunned, miserable, red-eyed faces to our concerned-looking waiter.

We're an annoyingly polite family at the best of times – only ordering starters once it's been ascertained that everybody wants one, filling DVD rental trips with the kind of no-you-choose routine that makes the process of selecting a movie longer than the film itself – but that day more than ever it was impossible to ascertain what anyone wanted to eat, so floored were we by the further details of my diagnosis. I took the reins again, hurriedly ordering nondescript plates of bravas, croquettas and tortilla, in an attempt both to get everyone sufficiently fed and to quickly shoo away our increasingly confused waiter.

Our roles, I realised, had reversed: suddenly I was the parent, taking care of my lost-looking, infantile brood; dishing out the don't-worrys and it'll-be-okays that I hoped would comfort them. Dad later admitted that he feared I was becoming our family's matriarch at such a young age. And, notoriously bossy as I am, it wasn't a position I was interested in. Almost as soon as the words 'breast cancer' had entered our world, it felt as if everyone was suddenly looking to me for strength and guidance and cues on how to act or what to say. And half of me felt pleased that they did; but the other half felt like a clueless, desperate child. What made anyone think that at twenty-eight – *twenty-eight!* – I was any better equipped than them to deal with this? Why was *I* suddenly the ringleader? *I* was the child. *I* was the one in trouble. *I* was the one in need of help. How could I scream my parents into submission one minute and expect them to wipe away my tears the next? Nothing, nothing, not a single fucking thing about this was fair, and I wanted to wail and scream and throw a noisy, fist-banging fit on the restaurant floor. But just as having to keep it together for everyone I loved wasn't fair, it was simultaneously the only thing I could bring myself to do.

When our crapas eventually arrived, I encouraged P, Mum and Dad to eat something, using their fork-pushing as an excuse to ignore my own food and instead make a list of the people I needed to keep informed. Jamie was first, then my mate Tills.

'Perhaps I ought to tell J,' said Mum.

'No, this is for me to do,' I snapped, in the manner of a haughty headmistress. 'In fact, I'm doing it right now,' I insisted, grabbing my phone from the table as though it were a clipboard from which I was about to read the school register. I stood watching P and my folks stare at their plates from the opposite side of the road as I called Jamie, picking at the flaking paint on some iron railings as his phone rang.

'Mate, it's me . . . it's invasive,' I revealed, wishing as soon as I'd said it that I'd found a better way to break the news.

'Fuck,' came the instant reply. 'Shit, sis . . . fuck. What are they going to do?'

I recounted the routine like a shopping list. 'Well, first I'm seeing a fertility expert to see whether I can get any eggs frozen before chemotherapy shoots the lot of them to shit. Then this Friday I'm having a mastectomy and once I've recovered from that there'll be a few months of chemo.' The phone line crackled with sniffs and mumbled expletives, but I continued with my cancer-catalogue. 'And then there'll be some radiotherapy and finally some hormone therapy, but to be honest I'm not really sure what that means.'

Jamie composed himself. 'And all of that is going to work, right?' I could sense the panic in his voice and it frightened the hell out of me.

'It'd fucking bett . . . yes, mate, of course it's going to work,' I corrected myself, choosing then and there to keep my doubts to myself. 'They're all really positive, J,' I said, finally finding a more sensitive tone. 'I'm young enough and tough enough to be able to handle this, y'know, and they're throwing everything they've got at it.'

I glanced back over to the restaurant window, trying to lip-read what P, Mum and Dad were saying to each other. I assumed this was a tapas-sized taster of what was to come: being talked about whenever I was absent, but continually unaware of what was being said.

'Will you be okay, dude?' I asked Jamie.

'Of course I'll be okay, you nobhead,' he replied, as I welcomed the relief of someone finally lightening the tone. 'I just want *you* to be, sis.'

My call to Tills went a similar way. I came clean about my tumour and recited the treatment shopping list. She gasped in all the right places and said 'fuck' a lot. Tills had clearly been steeling herself to hear the worst, and immediately switched into super-practical mode, deciding who she would tell on my behalf and how she could clear her diary for any time I might need her. She was brilliantly frank, and I was instantly grateful.

'I can't be doing with tears right now, Tills,' I said.

'Which is why you won't be getting any from me,' she replied. 'In fact, it's your duty to tell people to shut the fuck up whenever you want to. You've got to do this your way and it's not going to help if people are blubbering around you.'

I told her how I'd screamed my family into silence at the hospital, and she congratulated my efforts. 'That's my girl,' she said. 'You kick some ass.'

It seemed that there'd been some similar ass-kicking in the restaurant – though I'm still not sure by whom. By the time I'd made my calls and returned to my stool, P and my folks were sitting upright and feigning smiles, having apparently decided that straightforward and practical was their best tactic from here on in.

'We've been talking,' said Dad, 'and if you two want any time on your own, just say the word and we'll piss off back up the motorway.'

'That's more like it,' I thought to myself. Dad saying 'piss' and Jamie calling me a nobhead was exactly the kind of discourse I was after. Yes, this was The Worst News In The History Of The World, and yes, it was heartbreaking and upsetting and frightening and going to take one hell of a joint effort to get through, but there wasn't a hope of any of us getting through it if there wasn't even a sniff of light-heartedness about the situation.

'Yeah. I think maybe you'd better piss off.' I winked at Dad, turning to P for his consent. (As if he'd have disagreed. I'm sure if I'd have played Veruca Salt and asked for a pony and an MX5 and a Mulberry handbag he'd have let me get away with it.)

We paid our bill, piled into the car and headed back to the flat, making further lists of who to tell and how, each of our phones chirping a chorus of text-message beeps on the way. But as everyone else kept to their secret pact of staying practical and helpful and upbeat, our roles began to shift again, and I became the needy, petulant child to their calm, considered guardians. Bottom lip protruding, I stared out of the window at the backpacked tourists wandering along Baker Street, seeking out other girls my age. 'Why wasn't it you?' I thought as we passed a happy-looking twenty-something, arm in arm with her equally – and nauseatingly – happy-looking boyfriend. 'Why haven't *you* got this?'

I imagined all the things she could have done to justify a tumour in her breast. Perhaps she'd once seriously assaulted someone or committed fraud or perhaps her boyfriend was blissfully unaware of the husband and kids who assumed she was out at work. I made a mental list of the things I'd done that could have tipped my own karma in the wrong direction, but drew blanks at teenage hair-pulling, exaggerating my CV and stealing a carpet from an Indian restaurant in Freshers' Week. But even if I had nicked every CD in my collection, kicked the crap out of my school nemesis or cheated on every boyfriend I'd had, would that mean that I deserved to get cancer?

'It's not fucking fair,' I whinged when we got back home and resumed our positions – P on a floor cushion, me on the sofa, Dad in the armchair and Mum on the ottoman in the bay window. I wasn't timid or tearful or frightened. Just angry. Blood-boilingly angry. I needed to stomp and shout and swear and punch things – and I needed to do it on my own. So, selfish as it was to make them do it, my parents packed their car and drove back up to Derby, to give my brother the support he needed as much as any of us, and to

31

make arrangements to waste their annual leave on seeing me through The Bullshit.

My phone was ringing off the hook. Everyone had known that I was heading back to hospital for the details of my diagnosis, and the callers were a mixture of those curious to know the extent of my illness and those who'd just heard the grade-two-or-three reality. I ignored them all, choosing instead to tidy up the kitchen, throwing plates loudly and carelessly back into their drawers and kicking cupboard doors shut. Meanwhile P played secretary, cutting short every ring of my phone but eventually accepting a conference call from my bosses.

Hanging up the phone, P timidly explained what had been said: that work had signed me off immediately and that if ever there was anything they could do to help – taxis to the hospital, rescue packages, magazine subscriptions – to make sure they were the first people we called. Few companies would be so supportive, but not even their show of generous assistance could penetrate my blind rage. I was growing more livid with every second; more enraged with every breath. Hurling open my wardrobe doors and tearing bin liners off a fast-unravelling roll, I set to the task of pulling my newly bought summer clothes from their hangers, violently stuffing them into bags in protest at the summertime fun I would now be absent from.

Once my tantrum was done, P held me in his comforting arms, calming me with cuddles as the doorbell rang. My friend Ali had driven over, armed with cake, to do what she could to console us. She usually bursts in like the Tasmanian Devil, but this time she was quieter than usual as she edged around the front door and took herself into the kitchen to make a round of tea. P and I silently acknowledged what a huge deal it must have been for her to make this visit, having lost her mum to the same disease. 'Right then,' she said, positioning herself between us on the sofa. 'I've got something that'll cheer you up.' She produced from her pocket her mobile phone, pressing play on a series of hen-night-karaoke-session videos that I'd hoped P would never see. 'Whatever state this thing gets you into, Mac,' said Ali – one of the few people who still calls me by my maiden-name-influenced nickname – 'It can't be worse than this.' She pulled me closer for a one-armed hug as the three of us cried with laughter at footage of me rapping as well as a gin-fuelled Midlander is able.

'You bastard,' I said, nudging her with my shoulder. 'Don't you know I've got cancer?'

CHAPTER 4

The longest day

It's summer solstice, the longest day of the year. I've been up for little over an hour and already I know that this is the bleakest, lowest, blackest, most miserable day of my life.

Last night I sent my parents back up the motorway, thinking that P & I needed time alone. And it turns out we do need it, but actually with the safety of knowing that they're around too, fussing in the background. We're heading up to theirs as soon as I've published this blog post.

Today I'm struggling to locate my fighting force. I literally cannot cope. I've probably said that sentence some time before – perhaps after the deaths of my dear Nan and Grandad . . . revising for my A levels . . . just before the play-off final . . . or when I discovered my boyfriend in bed with his ex. Whenever I've said it before, it wasn't true. I *did* cope then. Right now I'm just not.

I find myself actually looking forward to surgery next week. I WANT THIS THING OUT OF ME. Cut me open, take my nipple, take the lot, scar me right up. Just get. it. out.

As terrifying as it seemed yesterday, right now I want to be in chemo, feeling like shit and losing my lovely long hair.

ANYTHING must be better than being in the midst of this dark, pathetic, can't-do-anything-about-it bullshit. But my hair and my tit can go now, and the sooner the better, because that'll mean that something's getting fixed.

*

Having gone to bed giggling the night before, it's probably no surprise that the reality came back to bite us on the ass the following morning. And boy, did it hurt. Our Saturday-morning routine normally involves the kind of duvet-based fun that my nineteen-year-old self would have rolled her eyes at: tea and toast in bed, newspapers, *Saturday Kitchen* on the telly and a cheeky bit of T-Rex before going shopping for that night's dinner ingredients. It's a lovely little custom – morning glory at its finest – and P and I are unapologetic about it being our favourite moment of the week. This Saturday, however, was different. Just as you wake up the first time after learning of a loved one's death, the devastating reminder of my invasive tumour shook us awake, trespassing on our marital bed, not even allowing us that blissful split-second of ignorance before the horrible weight of reality crushes you beneath its iron duvet. It was as though cancer was punishing us for not appreciating its gravity the night before.

I cried immediately after waking. 'I don't want to do this,' I whimpered into P's naked shoulder. 'I don't think I can.' I looked up to see his beautiful face wet with tears.

'But you must,' he croaked. 'You must. You must. You must. You must . . .' He wept more with every command and I realised for the first time that it wasn't just me who'd had this diagnosis – it was *us*: Me *and* P. Team Lynch. We were always ready to catch whatever was thrown our way. But this? This wasn't a gas bill or a gazumped flat or even another miscarriage. This had the potential to ruin it all. To put an end to me and P. To cut short our flawless marriage to a mere eighteen months. We howled loudly and messily into one another's pillows, grasping onto each other's bare skin as though letting go would mean admitting defeat so soon.

I threw back the sheets and staggered into the living room, hanging my head out of the window for air as though suffocated by the grief that was swallowing up our bedroom. Early-morning June sun peeped cheerily around the clouds, seemingly sticking its middle finger up at me and my life-endangering problems. The curtain rail wobbled precariously as I angrily swept the drapes back shut, furiously declaring to the world outside, 'This is the worst moment of my life.'

Look what it had done to us. Look what it was doing to our Saturday-morning routine. How fucking dare it. And look what it was yet to do – bursting our newlywed bubble, stealing a necessary part of my body then ruining what was left, forcing awful memories upon us, robbing us of our optimism. But most of all, this was supposed to be *our* time. How dare this thing encroach on our perfect, perfect time?

The fumes of our shattered morning left us unable to breathe. We had to get out. Throwing what we could into a holdall, we joined the travelling weekenders on the M40, tearing up the motorway to a place where, at least, there'd be someone to make us tea and run us a bath – the simple tasks we were suddenly incapable of doing. Mum and Dad were at the door to meet us, with Jamie and his fiancée Leanne two sheepish steps behind; all four of them doing what they could to disguise red eyes.

'I'm doing dinner tonight,' said Jamie.

'As if you hadn't suffered enough,' added Dad, his characteristic teasing concealing a broken heart. Jamie and Leanne pushed everyone aside to envelop me with hugs;

the kind of hugs that last a few seconds too long; the kind of hugs that suggest they're worried they might lose you.

'Meh,' I said, rubbing each of them on a shoulder by way of both comforting them and playing down the situation's seriousness. 'This is all going to be fine. Now, who's making me a brew?'

In another conversation I hadn't been party to, a plan of attack had clearly been agreed to keep this night as jovial as possible. Jamie was his usual hilarious self, turning Jamie Oliver to make chicken skewers and batting away Mum's interferences with a sarcasm that suggested she never used her kitchen herself. Leanne talked about her forthcoming nuptials, making bets on whether she or Jamie would come off worst from the hen/stag weekends. I suggested that, since I'd be bald for their ceremony, perhaps I should go for some laughs and give my reading in a funny accent, too.

We ate our chicken and reminisced about childhood memories. Of Jamie entering a talent show as a Michael Jackson impersonator, then collapsing into tears when he took the stage. Of the many mornings at Nan and Grandad's house, making tents beneath clothes horses, creating crazy golf courses in the garden and picking trodden-in Play-Doh out of the carpet. And of the time Mum left me on the potty to answer a phone call, only to wonder where I'd got the chocolate that was smeared around my mouth when she returned. Leanne's eyes almost burst out of her head; she was the only person in the room who hadn't previously been aware of my filthy secret. Ordinarily I'd be in bits about such an admission, but on that day my folks got away with it. Because, even if it took the revelation of my shit-eating, this was as good an example as any of my wonderful family's ability to crack a joke in *any* situation – and, by 'eck, was I grateful.

CHAPTER 5

New balls, please

The day before a mastectomy ought to be nervy and fretful and can't-eat-anything worrying. But I've never been one for doing things the right way around. Instead, I've spent the day before *my* mastectomy staring at Rafael Nadal's arse.

A particularly canny ex-boss with friends in all the right places had clearly anticipated that Mastectomy Eve had the potential to be a horribly squeaky-bum day, and thus wangled two front-row, number-one-court Wimbledon tickets for P and I, as a means of taking our minds off tomorrow's boob-removal. And what a terrific distraction it proved to be.

By 'it', of course, I mean Rafa's beautiful behind. Round, honed, perfectly peachy. You could sink your teeth into it. If you'd spotted me on the TV coverage, you'd have noticed that mine was the only transfixed head not following the ball from one side of court to the other. I became almost as obsessed with Rafa's bottom as I have recently with other people's boobs. I'm not ogling them, mind you – it's research. (And girls, that's the one time in your life when you can believe that line.) It was bound to happen. With all the chest-talk of late, I've quickly become a mammary meister. But seriously – when it comes to my new-look chest, will I be the Elephant Woman?

I worked myself up into a panic about that yesterday, while P and I snogged our way round London on an open-top bus (his tactic to divert my attention from tomorrow's inevitable). Will he still fancy me after the mastectomy (man, I hate that word), when I'm all stitched and swollen and unnatural-feeling and *sans* nipple? And, more to the bloody point, will he still fancy me when I'm pale and hairless, and bloated from the steroids? So lovely is P that he's offered to shave his head when my hair falls out. But I've told him not to – he's so darned handsome it'll ruin his looks, and I like him the way he is. And how ridiculous is that, eh?

*

'If one more person tells me to be strong,' said P on the morning of my mastectomy as we drove to the fertility clinic, 'I'm going to use what little is left of my strength to strangle the motherfucker.' I giggled, relieved that we were somehow able to turn our situation into an in-joke, just for us. But P's frustration was bang on the money. All we'd heard for the past few days was 'be strong', 'hang in there', 'stay positive', 'you can do it' . . . and to say it was doing our heads in was as much of an understatement as saying that I'd rather not lose my hair.

Once the initial shock settles in (which is a fib in itself, since it never really settles in) people's reactions naturally turn from stunned to helpful. But there are, of course, varying degrees of helpful. To me, helpful was being sent books and magazines and DVDs. Helpful was being given front-row tickets to Wimbledon. Helpful was not being treated any differently; not being looked at with a tilted head; not being thought of as a patient. (To this day, I still inflict death-stares on anyone who dares show purposeful concern about how I'm feeling. Even a simple 'are you all right, love?' has me itching to exact revenge with an evil Jedi mind trick.) And helpful was definitely *not* urging me to 'stay positive' (as though I hadn't considered that option already), and meeting my cancer news with the baffling 'I'm sure you won't let it beat you'. ('You're sure? Because, I've got to admit, I'm on the fence.')

But therein lies The Trouble With Cancer #1: however well-meaning or frustrating or enlightening or pointless or thoughtful their words may be, nothing anyone says can change the fact that you've got cancer. I don't want to sound like an ungrateful bitch here – even 'don't let it beat you' is better than saying nothing at all. And by no means am I suggesting that I've got a perfect record in reacting to other people's shitty news. I mean, who *does* know what to say in those situations? As a teenager, I took a call from my then boyfriend's mum to tell me the horrible news that his dad had died. I didn't know what to say. I said I couldn't believe it. I said I was sorry. And then, inexplicably, I asked if she needed any milk. Because the correct reaction to someone's husband dying is, of course, 'Shit, what if she can't make a brew?'

And so, you see, I'm the last person to be giving a lecture on the right way to react to bad news. Which brings me on to The Trouble With Cancer #2: the answer to what's best to say is, of course, different for everyone. Some people might want to be ignored. Some may want fawning sympathy ('poor you, must be awful'). Some might prefer outright anger ('I can't fucking believe this is happening to you'). But what did I want? Well, of all the messages I received, anything that was quietly understanding ('love you, thinking of you, no need to reply'), funny ('don't worry, sis, I'll visit you on the weekends . . . well, as long as Derby aren't playing at home') or put gossip above cancer ('someone just told me that Cher gets her arse vacuumed') pretty much hit the spot.

But of all of the reactions to my bullshit news, my favourite by far was from an ex-colleague. 'Breast cancer?' he said, stunned. 'That's awful . . . you've got such magnificent breasts.' (Applause.)

'And they'll be magnificent again,' I told him, more for my own benefit than his. Because, much as I'd convinced myself that losing a boob was nothing on losing my hair (which is faintly ridiculous, when you think about it), I'd have been lying if I'd said that I was anything less than terrified about the removal of my beautiful left tit.

The days prior to my op had thankfully been so filled with activity that I'd barely had time to fart, let alone reflect on what I was set to lose. But after waking up that morning to a breakfast of tears instead of toast, followed by brave face instead of bran flakes, it had suddenly become all too real. Before pulling on my black-and-white checked dress (I didn't think colourful florals were appropriate for such an occasion), I stood topless in front of my bedroom mirror. 'So this is it, then,' I whispered to my favourite boob. 'It's time for you to go.' And, fumbling with numb fingers to button up my outfit, that was the last I saw of my left tit. I didn't look down while my surgeon drew on his pre-op markings. I didn't catch a peek from the corner of my eye when changing into my hospital gown. I left it behind right there and then, as though waving it off on a station platform without turning back as the train pulled away.

'Bloody hell, this is posh,' said P as we pulled up outside the front door of the grand, Victorian fertility clinic on Harley

Street. The surgeon who'd diagnosed me had referred us here, assuring us that the expert we were about to see was our best chance of helping us freeze my eggs before chemo blasted them into obliteration. Uncomfortable in such imposing surroundings, we did our best to disguise our northern accents when checking in with the receptionist, minding our p's and q's and sitting up straight in the oak-panelled waiting room that looked more like a private school headmaster's office than a holding room for fertility-challenged couples.

'You must be Mr and Mrs Lynch,' said the Egg Man (which wasn't difficult to deduce, given that we were the only people in the waiting room). We nodded, following him into another equally impressive room and listening intently as he explained that time was of the essence, and that our best shot at gathering suitable eggs would be for me to have a course of hormones to boost their production. 'But all of this is hypothetical right now,' explained the Egg Man, looking up from a desk so huge you could have played snooker on it. 'It all depends on what the professor learns about the nature of your tumour later on today.'

P furrowed his brow to match mine. 'Sorry, um, I'm not – we're not . . .' he began, in a purposeful, alien voice that disguised his Liverpool roots. (The question in his head, I assumed, was, 'What the frig are you on about, la?')

'Depending on the histology results, the professor may decide, for instance, that it's safe to delay your chemo-therapy by a few weeks in order to have this course of hormones,' continued the Egg Man, unconsciously mark-ing dots on his notepad with a Biro. 'That's assuming the tumour is only where we believe it to be. And then there's the matter of whether or not the tumour is hormone receptive. If so, it might not be sensible to pump you full of oestrogen if that's what's caused the problem in the first place.'

'Well, no,' I agreed. 'So, then – let me get this straight. If my cancer is oestrogen receptive, I shouldn't have the hormone treatment. And if it isn't, we can go ahead with it.'

'Provided the tumour is only where we believe it to be,' he repeated.

'Well, yes. Right,' I said, superstitiously tapping his wooden desk. 'And how will you find this out?' I asked, more concerned about inter-hospital administration than the actual histology report.

'The professor will ring me with the result.'

'That's okay then,' I concluded, satisfied that the critical details of my tumour weren't being sent to him via carrier pigeon or telepathy or somesuch.

'I can't think about any of that shit right now,' I said to P as we made our way from the fertility clinic to the hospital. 'There's just no room in my head.'

He moved his hand from around my waist to the small of my back – as he did on the day of my diagnosis, as he always does when trying to protect me – and said, 'That's fine, babe. One thing at a time, eh?' I grabbed his hand tightly as we walked up the ramp to the hospital entrance, wheeling behind us the suitcase that we'd normally take on romantic weekend escapes.

Before showing me to my room, my professor's nurse introduced me to the sister on my ward. 'This is Lisa,' she said. 'She's here for her mastectomy.'

A frown appeared over the top of her spectacles as Sister looked suspiciously from my face to my bust, as though we might have been having her on about the breast cancer. I knew the look in her eye. The 'but she's so young' look. I'd later come to see that same look in the oncology clinic and the chemo room and the wig shop. 'Oh,' she said, devoid of emotion. 'I see.'

Clocking the potential awkwardness of the situation, my nurse quickly led me away, changing the subject with talk of how, prior to my op, she'd be accompanying me and Prof – I loved how she called him 'Prof' – to a clinic round the corner so that I could be injected with the radioactive dye that would determine whether the cancer had spread to my lymph nodes (known in the trade as a 'sentinel node biopsy', fact-fans).

'So how are you feeling?' Prof asked, as the three of us climbed into a people carrier that was parked outside the front of the hospital.

'Oh, y'know.' I grinned. 'I'm fine. Great.' I smiled a little wider, wondering whether it was the dread that was forcing me into being so cheery, or the fact that this man was about to remove from my body the tumour that was threatening to see me off before I'd even hit thirty. Probably the latter, I figured. (Hell, if you can't be nice to the man who's about to save your life, you've got to wonder whether your life is worth saving at all.) 'How's *your* week been, anyway?' I asked, keen both to force normal conversation and to suck up to my surgeon. 'Have you been working every day?'

'Oh, not every day,' he said. 'I had a day at Wimbledon this week.'

'Ooh! Me too! I went yesterday!' I squealed. 'Who did you see?'

'Ladies.' He paused. 'I can't understand why they grunt like that,' he said, as I basked in the appreciation of being able to enjoy a chat about grunting tennis players immediately before the most worrying event of my life. 'There really is no anatomical reason why they need to do it,' he continued. 'It's off-putting, don't you think?'

I nodded emphatically. 'Absolutely,' I concurred. 'Ab. So. Lutely.' (I suspected I'd have been agreeing with him just as forcefully if he'd suggested removing my breast with an ice-cream scoop, or that chopping off my left leg would improve my chance of survival.)

'And you? Who did you see?' he asked, turning his head to acknowledge me on the back seat.

'I saw Nadal,' I told him. 'It was brilliant. We had such a fantastic time. My old boss gave us the tickets in the hope that it would take our minds off today.'

'And did it?' he wondered, raising his eyebrows.

'Definitely,' I said.

'Well, that's good.' He smiled. 'And have you felt okay for the rest of the week?'

I glossed over the tears and the tapas and the terror, instead telling him that the past few days had been 'weird'. I joked that breast cancer had so far felt like having a *Groundhog Day* birthday, complete with wonderful gestures, breakfast in bed, cards, calls, letters, gifts, flowers, vouchers, cakes, visitors, chocolates, drawings from kids and a seahorse-shaped helium balloon.

'You've got a good team around you, then,' he replied, still smiling.

'Yep. At home *and* at the hospital,' I said, narrowly resisting the urge to wink.

The three of us continued to exchange beams and banter at the clinic as the professor drew markings on me in blue pen – one circling my soon-to-be-deceased nipple where he'd be accessing the inside of my breast, another underneath my armpit where he'd be collecting the sample of lymph nodes for my mid-op biopsy, and a final six-inch-long oval on my back, where he'd be taking some muscle that would form the basis of my new surgery-crafted tit.

'You're doing really well,' he said as he injected my underarm with radioactive dye.

I blushed, making as many dumb jokes as the situation allowed in the hope of coming across as girly and grateful rather than terse and terrified. The nurse gave me a caring rub on the shoulder as she helped me into my dress before we headed back to the hospital. 'Here we go, then,' I said with a shrug as we waited for the lift, the nurse and professor both staring at me with what I could only assume was compassion in their eyes.

'We were talking about you yesterday,' said my professor in his surgery gear, gesturing to the nurse as he pushed the button to the ground floor. 'And I have to say, I'm so impressed with how you've handled all of this so far.' My eyes widened and tears took their cue to form as he continued, 'I wish I could be more like you.'

Astonished by his compliment, I lost the power of speech. 'Pfah!' I exhaled, incomprehensibly. 'Wha . . . well, hah.' He continued to smile at me as I made a prize twat of myself. 'Crikey, well, I don't know about that,' I eventually retorted, my inability to know what to do with a compliment showing no signs of improving. I shuffled about uncomfortably, muttering 'thank you' and feeling grateful when the lift doors opened. Every time I've since relived that moment in my head – which is, at the last count, precisely 693, 821 times – I'm far cooler than I was in reality, playfully nudging his shoulder with a wink and an, 'Aw, I bet you say that to all your patients.' But, goofy as I was at the time, I couldn't escape the feeling of smugness that the man I was fast coming to hold in such sky-high esteem had said that *he* wanted to be more like *me*. It was like getting a report card filled with As, and I make no apologies for lapping up my opportunity to become teacher's pet.

Back on the ward, P, my folks and Jamie were waiting around the bed that was to become my base for the next five days, doing what they could to make my room feel less like a hospital and more like a student dorm: P tucking in a teddy bear, Mum tending to flowers, Dad setting up an iPod docking station, and Jamie blu-tacking a Foo Fighters greeting card that opened out into a phwoar-tastic poster of Dave Grohl. I changed into my gown and squeezed my calves into DVT socks, recommending some swanky local shops they might like to visit during the six hours I was expected to be in theatre. It was stupid, really – pretending that they'd be out on a jolly shopping trip rather than biting their nails to the bone until such a time as I was wheeled back to them – each of them was as frightened as me, and avoidance of the issue seemed like the best – if not the only – tactic.

'Are you ready to go then, darlin'?' asked a head that popped round the door.

'Ready as I'll ever be.' I shrugged. 'Come on, then,' I said, glancing over to my fraught-looking parents. 'Let's do this thing.' My bravado didn't last long – barely enough time for Mum, Dad and Jamie to kiss me and tell me that they loved me – for by the time I was wheeled out to the lift, gripping P's hand all the while, I was already in tears. My eyes burned with pure fear as I begged a higher force to let me wake up with this *thing* – this *bastard thing* – successfully removed from my body, never to return again. I looked nowhere other than into P's beautiful eyes – even as I was introduced to the anaesthetist – thinking that, if I wasn't going to survive this, they would be the last thing I'd wish to see.

'Have you had a general anaesthetic before?' asked the anaesthetist. I shook my head, still weeping. 'Well, there's nothing to worry about,' he continued. 'It'll just be like having a few G&Ts.'

My head answered, 'I could do with one of those,' but I didn't have the energy to articulate the thought, so fixated was I on my husband's loving face as the needle entered the back of my hand.

And then, with one too many shots of Gordon's, I was asleep.

CHAPTER 6

The equaliser

Ah, morphine. I'm whizzed off my tits.

I mean tit.

And, in the drug-induced spirit of everything being lovely, here's a thing to melt your heart. I just found the following text on my husband's phone (I may be flat out in a hospital bed, but I'm still sneaky enough to check people's phones when they're not looking): 'I know this is a strange message to send to my mother-in-law, but I've just seen your daughter's left breast and it looks amazing.' And I thought the morphine was good.

I might have a discoloured, odd-looking, wonky mound of flesh for a left tit, a strapless-top-restricting scar on my back and a catheter full of green wee (it's the dye, not the asparagus) but it's all for good reason: ding dong, the lump is dead!

But, in the bonfire-pissing spirit of cancer, there's bad news, too: accompanying my left tit in a hospital waste bin (I'm assuming) are the lymph nodes from my left armpit. The lot of them. That big bad bitch of a tumour had crept up a considerable way into my underarm (we'll find out how far later after some careful tracking on Google Maps or whatever it is they use), but thankfully my smiley, sent-from-heaven, superhero surgeon whipped them all out in one go. So, despite the setback, I reckon I can justifiably report that, in this match, I've just come from behind to score a wonder-goal of an equaliser (Smiley Surgeon with the blinding assist).

Lisa 1, The Bullshit 1. I'd do a celebratory Klinsmann dive, but I fear it might smart a bit.

*

'Still milking this breast cancer lark, then?' asked Jamie as he walked into my room the morning after my mastectomy.

'Piss off,' I retorted, grinning at him as he removed his jacket. 'Actually, J, Mum and Dad wanted me to keep this a secret from you, but I really think you ought to know that you were a mistake.' He winked at me as I beckoned him round to the other side of the bed. 'Seriously though, mate, just check this for me, will you?' I asked, pointing down towards the swamp-coloured catheter that was out of his line of sight.

'Sure, sis, what's th . . .? Oh jeez, you bitch,' he said in disgust upon seeing my bag of green piss. Jamie might be a big, manly, sport-obsessed geezer, but he's a squeamish one at that. I laughed as much as my painful chest would allow, threatening to show him my bloody wound if he continued to rib his sick sibling.

I'm always excited to see Jamie, but especially so on this day. Because, when you're bedridden and bruised, wearing this season's über-chic hospital gown in unfamiliar, worrying surroundings, with tubes seemingly coming out of every orifice, there is genuinely no better person to enforce some normality on the situation than Jamie. He really ought to hire himself out to people in these circumstances. Either that, or he should be on hospital radio. 'Suck it up, whingers,' he'd chirp, before playing 'Everybody Hurts', 'The Drugs Don't Work' or – for added shock-jock emphasis – 'Another One Bites The Dust'.

Our telephone call outside the tapas restaurant was the last serious talk Jamie and I had about cancer. To this day, every conversation between us that's involved The Bullshit has never been more than two strides away from humour. Even in the darkest moments of chemo, he'd delight in teasing me for being a hypochondriac, call me 'tit face' and insist to anyone who'd listen that the breast cancer was just another one of my attention-seeking tactics – all of which I'd let him get away with. For a famously close brother and sister like me and Jamie, not having a laugh with each other would have been as much of a tragedy as the breast cancer itself. Not just a tragedy, but plain *weird*. This wonderfully welcome piss-taking precedent was set the moment I was wheeled out from the theatre recovery room. Despite the expected post-op lethargy, when I first opened my eyes to see P and my family lining up outside my room, I found enough energy to give Jamie the middle finger before falling back into my morphine-assisted slumber.

What I didn't notice in that bird-flipping moment, however, was the relief etched on my family's faces, nor the tears that fell as I was being lifted from the trolley to my hospital bed. Because, while I was being unconsciously operated on, they had been busy tying themselves in worried knots. So in many ways, I had the easy job. After all, they were the ones who had to wander aimlessly around Central London as Smiley Surgeon cut around the outline of my nipple to access the tumour he spent an afternoon removing. They were the ones who forced themselves into time-occupying shopping missions (flowers, cards, a new charm for my bracelet, a lavender pillow to help me sleep) while my breast was replaced with a deflated, tissue-expanding temporary implant. And they were the ones who waited anxiously at the hospital, jumping at every noise, as my scheduled six-hour surgery sailed past the eight-hour mark. Sometimes, I guess, it's better to be the one in the shit than the one worrying about whoever's covered in it.

I don't remember a lot about the next few days in hospital, which is either to do with the on-tap morphine or the fact that it was so mind-numbingly boring – BBC Glastonbury coverage aside – that my brain immediately erased the lot, but what I do recall are the looks on the faces of my visitors as they sheepishly peered around my hospital door. It became clear that Jamie's teasing tactics weren't going to be everyone's style, and I could see that I was going to have to become skilled in figuring out within fifteen seconds of a visit how other people would want to play it. One friend immediately burst into tears, so I comforted her as best I could. Another's face drained of colour, so I offered him some of my many chocolates. Another was a terrifyingly animated version of her usual chirpy self. One mate's opening line was, 'Crikey, your hair looks good.' Another's was, 'All right, sicknote.' And another threw a packet of Monster Munch at me as he walked into the room.

Lovely as it was to be so inundated with well-wishers, it was my first taste of feeling like a museum exhibit; a freak-show to be viewed in single-file. (Roll up, roll up, for the one-breasted woman!) But rather than play the part of the ill person or feel conscious about my new, wonky-looking chest, I gave the people what they wanted, patting my non-tit whenever it was mentioned, waving around the drainage bottles that were collecting the excess blood from my wounds, and cracking as many cancer jokes as I could (the aforementioned 'whizzed off my tit' became my personal favourite). It made me feel better. It made them feel better. And it was the best weapon I had in my cancer-beating arsenal.

During one visit, though, the jolly stuff didn't come quite so easily. It was the afternoon after my surgery when Smiley Surgeon first came to see me, and it was Mum's turn to be on keeping-me-company duty. In walked my hero, all beaming pleasantries and ear-wide smile, demonstrably pleased with his work.

'You look really well,' he said cheerily as he greeted me and Mum.

'Ha, cheers,' I blushed as Mum moved to stand beside my bed, offering him a captive audience for whatever it was he was about to say.

'So the operation went well,' he continued as we nodded along like two plastic dogs in a rear windscreen. 'However, the sentinel node biopsy showed a spread to your lymph nodes, so I removed them immediately,' he revealed.

I gulped, shooting a sideways glance at Mum, who was equally stumped for words. I wasn't shocked, necessarily. Hell, I was maxed out on shock – I reckon if he'd revealed that a blind work-experience volunteer had operated on me, I'd have stayed reasonably unruffled. Perhaps it was more disappointment. 'So it *did* spread,' I conceded calmly, though I'm not sure to whom.

'It did, yes.' He nodded. 'But I'm very optimistic. Remember, it has all gone now; it has all been removed. And the chemotherapy will mop up any rogue cells that are too small to operate on.'

As was fast becoming the case during these bombshell moments, I stopped listening, leaving it to Mum to ask questions and talk prognosis and histology reports (thanks to working in a hospital, she's down with that kind of language). While they talked, I tried to reason with the news in my mind. 'Let's look at the facts,' I told myself. 'First it was in my tit. Then it crept into my lymph system. But it's out now. It's gone. He's got rid of it. So yes, it's a bigger deal than you thought it was, but has it really made any difference? Did you even know what lymph nodes were before all of this? Would you be able to draw them in a game of Pictionary? No. So what the hell can they have been doing that's so vital to your well-being? Come on, now, people live perfectly long and fulfilled lives without a kidney, and you know what they're for. So what's a few lymph nodes between friends?' I dare say the industrial-strength painkillers helped with my sober reasoning, and Mum's relaxed insistence that it didn't matter to the outcome as long as the nodes had been removed freaked me out more for her enforced calmness than the news itself.

I appreciate that this is yet another stoically British way of looking at things, but, really, when the worst has happened, what does another setback matter? It's like getting soaked in the rain on your way home and then stepping in a puddle. Yes, it's a pisser, but can you really be arsed getting that worked up about it? I spoke about this with Ant recently, after which she likened me to one of those battleaxes that French and Saunders used to play – chopping off a finger by accident and feeding it to the dog, then slicing off another when the other dog looked hungry. 'Ah well, love, what's another finger?' she mocked.

The thing is, in the series of mini-battles that characterised my first few days in hospital, to me, the grade-three reality of my cancer was just another hurdle to jump. In the situation I found myself – with even sitting up straight or drinking a cup of tea seeming like a huge deal – all sense of perspective was launching itself out of my fourth-floor window.

For example, the day I managed to put on my pyjamas was a huge deal to me. This sounds pretty daft now I see it written down, but at the time, with the pain in my chest and back that I couldn't precisely locate and the stiffness that prevented me from moving my left arm properly, even bending my elbow to reach inside my pyjama sleeve was quite the achievement. (Not least because they won the prize for The World's Least Attractive Sleepwear. I'd only let Mum buy them because it made her feel better.) It was so much of an achievement, in fact, that it became the first in a series of triumphant cancer-milestone photos sent via media message from my mum to my brother, in which I'm giving him yet another middle finger. It's not your average family album, granted, but it's cherished nonetheless. ('There's Lisa in hospital, giving Jamie the middle finger. That's Lisa again, with the first meal she ate after chemo, giving Jamie the middle finger. And there's Lisa in her headscarf, giving Jamie the middle finger . . .')

Another goal was achieved the first time I walked down the ward corridor. Actually, waddled is a more accurate description. In fact, my first few steps were as far removed from a confident catwalk strut as you're likely to get, thanks to a baggier-on-the-left pyjama top and my having to shuffle about with a bag of drainage tubes on one side and a bag of piss on the other (Mulberry eat your heart out). You'd think it would have been the hospital-issue handbags that would have embarrassed me the most, and yet, when I spotted Tills and her husband Si at the other end of the corridor, my strange combination of joy at seeing them and shame at them seeing me was more down to my grandma-chic spotty pyjamas than the bottle of urine in my right hand.

But the biggest fence to jump came in an even more unsavoury form – and equally unsavoury surroundings: the toilet. The cancer, I was just about getting my head around. But the constipation? Shit! (Or no shit, as the case may be.) Sheesh, those leaflets they hand over on diagnosis should read, 'Welcome to breast cancer. Leave your vanity at the door and let's crack on, shall we?'

It's a simple equation, really. General anaesthetic + loads of drugs = an arse that's as tough to crack as the Enigma Code. And so, on my penultimate afternoon in hospital, I put a nurse through the unenviable task of shoving a suppository up my jacksie (at the end of her shift, poor cow!), and later watched P's best man wince as he was uncomfortably sandwiched in the middle of a mid-visit medical conversation about the softness of my stools. (Vanity? What vanity?) It's a good job P and I had married already, or that could have been some serious ammunition for his speech.

But after hardship, of course, comes relief. And later that evening, to the televised sound of 15,000 Wimbledon tennis fans on my hospital TV (and a coach-like husband willing me on from the other side of the toilet door), I produced my own Murray-esque fightback. 'Thank you, Wimbledon,' I said to myself in the mirror as I washed my hands. 'You were a wonderful crowd. I couldn't have done it without you.'

CHAPTER 7

Save Ferris

July 2008

Nobody ever enjoyed ill health (in particular the attention it brings) quite like my grandad. After having heart surgery, he spent the subsequent few years sitting in his chair breathing loudly, with a hand placed purposefully over his heart, just itching for someone to acknowledge it.

After my diagnosis, I joked that perhaps I could attract the same kind of attention by walking about with my hand constantly on my left tit. And ta-dah! Here I am, sitting in the chair beside my hospital bed, typing with my right hand while grabbing my prosthetic boob with my left. My left arm remains pretty screwed – to the point of not being able to tie my hair back and needing someone to dress me – so holding onto my prosthetic tit is as good a use as any for it, eh? Call it physiotherapy.

But yes, the falsie. Cancer really does get more glamorous by the day, I tells ya. Just as I was enjoying the joyful moment of being unplugged from my various wound drains before being discharged from my five-day hospital stay, in comes my very lovely (and always-bloody-right-about-everything) breast nurse to fit me for the bra that I must wear, day and night, until someone tells me otherwise. Believe me, this brassiere is no Agent Provocateur contender. But more of that later.

What the bra does have, however, is a handy little pocket to house the prosthetic boob that I'm currently sporting (keep an eye out for them next Fashion Week). It's round and foamy and stuffed with lambswool, and it feels a bit like a novelty clown's nose (honk honk). And while I'm thankful for it in the meantime so I don't have to look all wonky-chested in my high-necked clothes, I'll be more enthusiastic when we can eventually get round to the fun of inflating my currently flat saline implant. (That said, it'll be limited fun – it's only got my usual B-cup level to imitate, so we'll hardly be putting it to the Dolly Parton test.)

Speaking of inflation, there's been a weird side-effect on that front that I hadn't really bargained for. You've seen *Willy Wonka and the Chocolate Factory*, right? (The kinda crap '70s one, not the trippy Johnny Depp one.) Well, think of Violet Beauregarde filling with blueberry juice after eating that dodgy chewing-gum, and you've got a pretty good idea of how my left side has felt since my wound drains were taken out. Always-Right Breast Nurse warned that my skin 'might begin to feel like a filled-up hot-water bottle' and, true to form, she's not wrong. Fortunately Smiley Surgeon has got the Oompa Loompas on hand to drain me next week. And hopefully after that, this damn bra will become a bit more comfortable. Not that my newly deflated left side will make my cancer-patient lingerie look any more passable in the fashion stakes, you understand.

From a distance (the other side of a football field, let's say) it looks a bit like a training bra, or a cropped gym top (the really show-offy kind that you see those leathery women in their sixties wearing while jogging over Chelsea Bridge in rush hour). Up close, mind, it looks like something that could have had a previous life on my nan's washing-line. It's off-white (naturally, it doesn't come in any other colours) with wide straps and nondescript flowers embroidered onto it, the like of which you'd normally see on a naff B & B bedspread. This bra is all the proof you need that the medical world just ain't used to dealing with breast cancer in twenty-somethings. It is the anti-sexy. Poor P's already got bollocks like cricket balls and, with this lingerie look, it doesn't look like being remedied any time soon.

*

'Blimey, you're popular, ain'tcha?' said my cheery postie, handing over a wedding-day-worthy pile of mail at my front door as she had done most days since people started hearing about The Bullshit. The recurring birthday I'd joked about with Smiley Surgeon was showing no signs of slowing, particularly since I'd been home from hospital, and I struggled to keep up with the baffling tidal wave of niceness that was heading my way.

I couldn't believe the kind of things people were doing for me. Sending huge packages filled with things that might help, flying from abroad to visit, sorting out a car service to take me to and from my hospital appointments, calling Charles Worthington's PA to find out who he'd recommend to be entrusted with my pre-chemo, lop-off-the-length haircut . . . *ah-may-zing* stuff. I was half expecting to see my name on a blimp, in a newspaper headline or on a score-board at the baseball, Ferris Bueller-style.

It was all so staggeringly lovely – and a massive help to boot – but I struggled to figure out up to what point should I accept it? It's not like I wasn't milking my position when I had the chance, mind you. In fact, I was fast coming to realise that this illness seemed like the perfect excuse for absolutely any kind of behaviour whatsoever – and I was going to use it. Someone reluctant to give way on the road? I'd pull out first anyway: 'Fuck it, I've got cancer.' One slice of pizza left? 'Fuck you lot, I'm having it – I've got cancer.' It may have been a hopeless case of sifting for gold in a pile of dog poo but you've got to grab your fun where you can in times like these. But sometimes, even despite my enthusiasm to exploit cancer for all it was worth, the treatment I was receiving from other people was just so overwhelming that I felt compelled to make it stop.

When I'd question their kindness, they'd tell me that they were doing it because they loved me and that, if I weren't so nice in the first place, they wouldn't want to bother. But I worried that, actually, they'd got it all wrong, and that their spectacular efforts were wasted. Because the thing is, I'm really not always that nice.

I can be a real grumpy/selfish/bitchy/lazy/stubborn/ sensitive/manipulative/cheeky cow when I want to. I got the hump when Princess Diana died and ruined my eighteenth birthday. I hardly ever make a brew for my colleagues. I once used someone's office for a purpose other than work. I'm late for EVERYTHING. I've taken refunds on clothes that I've worn. I've cadged more fags than I've bought. I bunked more uni lectures than I went to, and made up poor excuses to get my deadlines extended. I continually correct people's grammar, and carry around a red pen to scrub out rogue apostrophes on posters/ menus/birthday cards.

I lie as well. I've been known to do it on my CV, but it's mostly in situations where I know it'll embarrass the arse off someone. Like the time I told P that OutKast were from Pontypridd, not Georgia, then watched as he tried to persuade other people of the same. Or when I called my brother in a rage, incensed that the New Year Honours list included a knighthood for Vernon Kay, in recognition of his charity work. (Sir Vernon Kay! I ask you! Apparently the more ludicrous the lie, the better the result.) Or in Freshers' Week when I began a rumour that I'd turned down a place in the Spice Girls to study for a degree. Or the day I told some kids at school that my dad was an ex-Derby County player. And then there was the night when my brother was having a house party, so I got my mate to call him up, pretending to be the police reporting a noise complaint. The result was magnificent: Jamie's mates have never let him forget it, and it still makes me feel fantastic. With a piss-taking history like that, it was a wonder anyone even believed the earth-shattering news from the girl who cried cancer.

It was a strange old time, the week after getting out of hospital. Suddenly, it seemed, The Bullshit wasn't a mere news story any more, but an actual, live-feed, twenty-four-hour event that everybody wanted to get in on. And it couldn't have felt more surreal. Back in my pre-cancer life, I'd hear the word 'cancer' and leap to all the assumptions that such an ugly word carries – that it must be excruciating; that it must make you feel horrific; that you'd obviously know you had it before you were even told. But, of course, it doesn't work like that. And, in the early stages at least, it's not the cancer that makes you feel so dreadful, but the treatment. And the treatment was what I had in store next.

The trouble was, I didn't *feel* like I had cancer. If anything, I felt like I'd had a bit of cosmetic surgery and, stitches and swelling and stiffness aside, I felt oddly fine. So, despite the fact that I had a disease that could kill me before I was thirty, I was queuing up episodes of *Coronation Street* on Sky+. And despite the fact that I'd had a life-threatening tumour growing beneath my nipple mere days before, I was busy filling my diary with pre-chemo lunches, pub visits and dinner parties with my mates. In fact, I was more popular than I'd ever been. Breast cancer, it seemed, had made me interesting.

Which was strange, because I'd always felt rather uninteresting. If my school had created a yearbook, I'd have been the Girl Most Likely To Have A Normal Life, and I appreciated and objected to that in equal measure. I'd always done everything exactly as it was expected of me; exactly as I'd planned it. GCSEs by sixteen. A levels by eighteen. Bachelor's degree by twenty-one. Master's degree by twenty-two. Magazine editor by twenty-five. Married by twenty-seven. All strictly by the book. No truancy, no shoplifting, no tattoos, no inappropriate piercings, no arrests, no unwanted pregnancies, no off-the-rails drugs binges, no havoc-filled gap years, no weekend-long illegal raves, no hopeless romances with a bad-influence bass guitarist (dammit). So had my lack of Drew Barrymore-esque, wild-child teens or reckless, selfish twenties somehow mutated into a rebellious tumour? As a kid, I'd adored the 'Solomon Grundy' poem. Was The Bullshit my 'took ill on Thursday'?

Don't get me wrong, I'd enjoyed all the foolish, unscheduled fun that a twenty-eight-year-old lass ought to be able to check off her list, and in the process earned my Brownie badges in tequila shots, one-night stands and puking from cab windows, but all of it had been done within the kind of perimeters that meant nobody got hurt. ('Fun with rules', as P would call it.)

I was happy with my life as it was. But I had occasionally wished I could be that little bit more interesting. Well, guess what? Now, I *was* interesting – but I didn't want any part of it. Lovely as it was to be getting so much ego-flattering attention, every now and then I'd remember the reason why I was getting it in the first place, and the reality would leap up to bite me on the ass like a rabid dog. Within seconds, I'd lurch from smugly arranging beautiful bouquets of flowers to collapsing into frustrated tears at the kitchen sink, alarmed that my treatment had got so swiftly underway and terrified about what it might have in store.

My treatment at the hands of cancer was, of course, the reason for my treatment at the hands of my friends and family. They were spoiling me with kind gestures because it was the only thing they could do. They couldn't take the cancer away, nor could they fraudulently endure the treatment on my behalf like some kind of twisted driving-test scam. But what they *could* do was let me know – on a scale grander than you'd ever experience at Christmas or on a birthday or at your wedding – just how much they loved me, and assure me that, whatever nasty surprises The Bullshit had lined up, they'd be there for me to fall back on; the safety net beneath my swinging trapeze.

CHAPTER 8

The no-kids clause

Smiley Surgeon and Always-Right Breast Nurse were on good form at my mastectomy-follow-up appointment today. They're right on my wavelength that, whatever news they have to deliver, it surely can't be worse than what they told me three weeks ago. Hence, they're always very chipper and matter-of-fact, and keen to talk tennis before cancer.

There was a great moment today when my dressings came off for the first time, and we were all able to admire Smiley Surgeon's handiwork. Man, that guy should set up an alterations business – his stitching is the nuts. I've got one slightly diagonal scar on my back that's about the length of a Curly Wurly, then one under my armpit that's a bit shorter than a KitKat finger (thankfully not the Chunky version). They're both super-neat and healing fast, and they won't be the kind of thing I'm embarrassed about being visible in the future. (Low-back tops are back on the shopping list. Or at least they would be if I could carry them off in the first place.)

But – drumroll please – the mother of all wounds is at the front. And what a corker it is. I've never been a tits-out-for-the-lads kind of girl, but now I might just become one. In my mind,

I had envisaged some sort of heinous, purple X-shaped gash with bruising all around it and stitches poking out at untidy angles, crusty blood still hanging off. (Enjoying your dinner?) In reality, though, my boob looks precisely like it should, considering what it's been through. In short, my nipple has been lopped off (technical term) and replaced with a graft of skin from my back. Imagine it all as a slightly-squashed oval shape with a circle the size of a Quality Street Toffee Penny in the middle, and you've got the picture. Not bad, eh? No wonder the four of us were cooing over it this morning. 'Tis a beautiful thing.

But onto the rest of the follow-up. (Consider all of the above 'talking tennis before cancer'.) Because the remainder of today's hospital visit concerned the serious stuff of histology reports and treatment timelines. So first, the good news:

1. Despite the tumour having pushed dangerously close to my skin, that biopsy came back clear. And, let's be honest, I could have done without skin cancer as well.
2. I'm healing quickly, in every sense. I shan't be doing the 'YMCA' for a while, but at least now I've got an excuse for being the miserable git who won't participate in a Mexican wave.
3. The tumour is gone. Next week's CT scan (that is worrying me more than I care to admit) will determine whether there is any further spread, but that bulky bitch of a lump that caused all this fuss in the first place is out.

And then the not-so-good news:

1. For a grade-three cancer, this is one aggressive motherfucker (Smiley Surgeon may have phrased that differently): it had spread to twenty-four out of twenty-five of my lymph nodes at what appears to be an

alarmingly fast rate. (I bet that twenty-fifth node was a right cocky bastard.) And so the upshot is, we've got to move fast on the chemo.

2. My cancer is more hormone-receptive than we might have thought. So the quick pre-chemo course of IVF as a means of ensuring that we've got options when it comes to having kids is now off the menu, as is any hope of freezing eggs prior to my next phase of treatment. We just can't hang around waiting for my ovaries to cough up the good stuff and risk my cancer spreading any further.

3. But that's not all. The hormone-receptive stuff could perhaps be, in one way or another, my fault. Almost exactly a year ago, I had the first of two miscarriages, so there's a chance that my getting pregnant in the first place could have exacerbated the cancer. (See, kids, SEX IS DANGEROUS.) There's no definite way of knowing whether or not either pregnancy was to blame for The Bullshit, but we cannot ignore the fact that they could have given it a leg-up. Either way, it turns out that oestrogen might just be my kryptonite.

*

I'm still baffled by the immediate way in which P and I reacted to the blow to our fertility. Much like the truth about cancer's spread to my lymph nodes, it felt rather like conceding a penalty when we were already ten-nil down. There was almost, dare I say, a dark comedy to it. I couldn't help but think about an exceptionally unlucky bloke I used to work with. If there was a hole, he'd fall down it. If there was broken glass, he'd step on it. If there was a burglar in his town, his house would get robbed. If there was a hooligan at a footy match, he'd be the one who got punched. So, rather predictably, he earned the nickname Lucky. And here we were: Mr and Mrs Good Fortune. First the miscarriages; then a lump; then cancer; then an aggressive spread; then fertility issues. Ha ha ha.

'I'm starting to wonder whether I might have been a Nazi leader in a former life,' I said to P as we lay side by side on our bed, staring at the ceiling in disbelief. 'Seriously. What can we possibly have done to deserve such a monumental run of bad luck? You haven't killed anybody and not told me, have you?'

P rolled onto his right side to get a bit closer. 'Not that I know of, love,' he said, resigned. 'But with all this happening to us I might yet. So much for sodding karma, eh?'

The thing was, with the looming, unknown prospect of chemotherapy a matter of days away, there just wasn't space in our heads to squeeze in yet another stomach-punching blow from The Bullshit, and so instead we kind of ignored it, with a 'well that's that, then' attitude, however ridiculous that might sound now. It's particularly ridiculous, I suppose, when you consider that pre-Bullshit, *everything* for P and I was geared towards having a baby.

But, the way we saw it, had we been told in the course of our post-miscarriage fertility checks that we wouldn't be able to have our own children, that would have been a genuinely gut-wrenching disappointment. We'd have cried and mourned for the kids we'd already named (Maisy Jean for a girl, Cameron Thomas Arthur for a boy) and immediately got our names on an adoption register. But now, things were different. Because, aside from the fact that this news was rather on the woolly side ('having kids could be dangerous to you' is an altogether different prospect to the straightforward 'you *can't* have kids'), there were bigger issues at hand. Y'know, like staying alive and stuff. Not to mention my much more time-pressing worries about what chemo would do to me . . . whether it would work, how it would make me feel and what it'd do to my looks.

I remember having a recurring dream in which, almost every night, a different boy I knew would learn that I had breast cancer. He'd then take an ill-looking me out on a date and, at the end of the night, kiss me meaningfully, as though he were trying to prove that he was cool with the C-word. Granted, this wasn't a nightmare – and it was a welcome change to my usual dream where I have to wait ages in the toilet queue of a busy club, only to find when I get to the front that the only available cubicle has no door – but I couldn't help but wonder whether it had something to do with my fear of becoming completely unfanciable when all the hair-loss and steroid-swelling fun began. Because – kids or no kids – *nothing* was more important to me than having P around.

One night that week, P jogged home from work. 'I'm taking my frustration out on the pavement,' he said, when I questioned the change from his usual method of commute. He mentioned that some girls sitting on a bench had commented on his legs. Of course they did. P is gorgeous. And clearly, I wasn't the only one to have noticed his charms (go near him and I'll scratch your eyes out, right?), which was something that came to play on my mind more than it might have done ordinarily. Actually, that's playing it down somewhat. I was completely bloody petrified that he was going to go off me. Because, let's be honest, balding, bloated lasses aren't most blokes' idea of a model wife, are they? And definitely not balding, bloated lasses who are unlikely to give them a child of their own.

All I was hearing from the sensible people around me was not to concern myself with what was around the corner; to deal with the present; to take each day as it came. But that was rather like asking a dog not to bark. Whether or not I communicated it, cancer's looks-destroying, fertility-sapping potential was occupying my thoughts more than I knew it should. And all I could think about was what a bum deal all of this was becoming for P. Was the no-kids stuff going to become a huge regret for him? Might he one day wish he hadn't woken me up at six o'clock that Thursday morning, with the promise of a wonderful life together and an enticing Tiffany box? And there was always going to be some bench-bitch with a compliment on his legs, ready to divert his attention from his once-beautiful bride.

I don't really know what it feels like to have major eat-away-at-you regrets. Mine are more like loose ends I wish I'd tied up when I had the chance. I wish, for example, that I'd been nicer to the very decent bloke I had a long-distance almost-relationship with following a couple of very fun dates in our home town, then gave the brush-off when he travelled miles to visit me in London (not because I didn't like him, but because I'd had my heart broken in the meantime and was frightened of getting close to another boy again). I wish I'd never lost touch with my dear friend Weeza, who missed out on my wedding as a result of our time apart – a fact that will upset me as long as I live. I wish I'd stood my ground in a particularly stressful former job, and done more to avoid the trouble it caused for me and my friends. And I wish I'd never shelled out my monthly travel budget on some unfeasibly high shoes I wore to a friend's wedding. Not only were they toe torture, they also gave me pins like Miss Piggy's and were never worn again.

But all of those things seemed like mere details in comparison to the regrets that P could later come to have about his choice of wife. At our wedding, we'd opted for different vows than the usual 'for better or worse, in sickness and in health' (luckily). Instead, we promised to care for each other with love and friendship; to support and comfort each other through good times and through troubled times; to respect and cherish each other and to be faithful always. But, on that spectacularly beautiful day in December – a mere eighteen months previous – neither of us could have imagined that those 'troubled times' might come to mean all of this.

Thanks to our duo of disappointingly short pregnancies, P and I had, of course, been forced to consider a life that included just the two of us. It mostly involves us watching cricket all over the world, lots of four-poster-bed weekends away, buying a second house in Spain, always going to Glastonbury in a pimped-up camper van, and owning a ridiculously child-unfriendly Zone 1 apartment with a massive roof terrace that's perfect for parties. Now, that's not a distant-second-place existence. I LOVE the thought of that life with P. (Jeez, I love the thought of *any* life with P. Stick us in a hut in Hull and we'd still have a good time.) And, even during the bleakest moments of The Bullshit, P would tell me that he felt exactly the same about our alternative future.

But, in that peculiar time of everybody treating me like a china doll, it was difficult to figure out when people were being honest, or avoiding the tricky stuff and instead telling me what they thought I wanted to hear. Even P. I'd bring up my concerns in as breezy a way as I could manage, and every time he'd bat them away like flies around his beer glass.

'Don't be so daft,' he'd protest, stroking my lovely long hair. 'You've got a gorgeous face – and that's not going to change, is it?'

'But what about the other stuff?' I'd ask. 'I'm not the wife you bargained for. Your life's hardly turning out the way you thought it would, is it?'

Then he'd dissolve my line of reasoning in an instant, the way only he can. 'You mean *our* life,' he'd say, locking his fingers with mine. 'We're in this together, remember?'

And I'd smile. And shut up. Because you just can't argue with that.

CHAPTER 9

The science bit

Let the games commence! I've been at the hospital all afternoon and have come out with so much new info that I feel like I've had a crash course in another language. The next time you get a difficult cancer question at the pub quiz, consider me your phone-a-friend.

Aware that today marked the entry point to phase two of The Bullshit, I made the emancipatory move of ditching my mastectomy bra for the first time, and proudly wore my wonky chest in a favourite top and bust-skimming pendant necklace with jeans and my I-can-take-anything-on-provided-it-doesn't-mean-walking-far wedges. Cancer may take my hair, but it'll never take my fashion sense.

I tottered precariously into the hospital and was handed a pristine-looking file with my name on it that had to accompany me up to a different floor. Being a nosy cow, I had a good look through it while waiting for the lift: it was divided into neat, currently empty sections like 'histology', 'chemotherapy reports' and 'radiotherapy reports'. As the lift doors opened onto my floor, I noticed two things: (1) not everyone's files were so pristine (apparently cancer treatment takes it out on you *and* your folder), and (2) I was the youngest person in the waiting room by about, ooh, a hundred years. My wedges were wasted on this lot.

After the routine up-the-nose MRSA test, in came The Cavalry, aka the curly-haired professor and his absolutely stunning second-in-command (she'll be a great help when I'm in full George Dawes mode – couldn't they have found me a troll-like consultant instead?). And they were both brilliant: the perfect mix of straight-talking without the scariness and empathetic without the head-tilting.

Curly Professor explained that, whatever the results of my CT scan, it would have no bearing on the chemotherapy I'd be having. Whether or not it actually revealed any further spread, he told me that it was best to assume that there *would* be cancer cells elsewhere in my body (thanks to so many lymph nodes being involved), which, oddly, came as quite a comfort. I had been completely cacking it before my scan (which is as close to the World's Biggest Understatement as you're likely to get), but hearing this did a lot to ease my worry. There's huge relief in knowing that, whatever the scan reveals, I'll be having the right treatment to zap the arse off it anyway.

All that said, my oncologists' serious looks made everything feel all too real. I wanted to stop them mid-flow and say, 'Hang on, now, let me get this right. I've got *breast cancer*? And you're about to give me *chemotherapy*? That's pretty fucking hard-core, no?' Up to now, it seems, all of this has been a comparative blast when you take a look at the months of toxic treatment ahead. What a bastard.

So here's the science bit: I'll begin with three sets of three-weekly cycles of one type of chemo, then have the same number of cycles of a different type. The side-effects that Curly Professor listed didn't exactly read like a menu of spa treatments, and Glamorous Assistant nodded along sagely throughout (actually, she did offer a conciliatory head-tilt at the hair-loss part, since her lovely curly locks rival even the professor's). Curly Professor was at great pains to point out that they'd be 'throwing everything at it', and that, thanks to my age and health, he intended to give me strongest dose of chemo possible. Then out came reams of consent forms to further enhance his point.

In better news, though, he agreed to fix my chemo cycles so that Jamie's wedding falls in my 'good week' (the third week of my cycle), so I can return the favour of dancing with him to an indie classic, and look as glamorous as is possible with no eyelashes and a wig.

Later at the hospital, there was my CT scan to keep my mind off the size of the chemo needles, and it was far more entertaining than it should have been. Lying on a moving bed in a futuristic white room while a tunnel-like machine scanned my body made me feel a bit like Kanye West in the 'Stronger' video (but wearing a nasty NHS gown instead of white boxer shorts). And even the injection during the scan was a bit of a giggle, thanks to its rather unusual consequences: since when has feeling like you've pissed yourself been an acceptable side-effect? It was the strangest thing, and pretty bloody embarrassing to boot. Just to clarify, I didn't *actually* piss myself. It just felt like I had. I'd like to be able to tell you that I've never pissed myself, but there was that regrettable little accident I once had on a ski slope in my salopettes, thanks to my snail-paced snowplough not getting me to the loo on time.

I got to have a quick look around the chemo room, too. And, I'll be honest, it was hardly soothing music, essential oils and people in fluffy white dressing gowns. But nor was it a scene from *The Exorcist*. Some poor sods looked pretty bloody poorly, but others looked like they'd just waltzed out of Selfridges. Ever keen to do things my way (or no way at all), I've decided not to be a cancer patient, but instead a mere guest who's booked herself in for a relaxing day in the Therapy Suite. I'm going to turn up in huge sunglasses, comfy jeans, a kick-ass T-shirt and my sparkly new Converse trainers, with my Marc Jacobs tote in one hand and my iPhone in the other, and completely ignore the real reason I'm there. Ladies and gentlemen, breast cancer just got fabulous.

*

'That's not like you,' said P as I stood in my knickers, straightening my hair at the foot of the four-poster bed in our magnificent hotel in the Ashdown Forest where we'd gone for our pre-chemo romantic night away. I furrowed my brow.

'Eh? How do you mean?'

'You. That,' he said, sprawled across the bed reading the newspaper in his complimentary robe. 'In your knickers. Parading around, uninhibited. Don't get me wrong, babe, I'm enjoying it. But it's just not like you, is all. Look, the curtains are even open.'

'Meh, it's only deer out there anyway.' I shrugged, but P had a point. It wasn't like me at all.

You see, I've spent as long as I can remember wishing I looked different. As a kid, I loathed my super-curly, strawberry-blonde (okay, ginger) hair. I was hardly blessed with a good set of gnashers either. In fact, that's another huge understatement, so I'll instead use the words of my dad, who chose his father-of-the-bride speech to announce that I had 'teeth like Ronaldinho'. At twelve, I convinced myself that I was the hairiest girl in the second year, and threatened to ring ChildLine when Mum refused to let me shave my legs. By thirteen, I had become quite obsessed

75

with the agonisingly slow rate at which my boobs were growing. (Turns out having tits isn't all it's cracked up to be.) By fourteen, it was all about the acne. At fifteen, I swore off short skirts on account of my wonky left knee. By sixteen, I was more concerned with the size of my arse (no change there). And ever since, it's been everything from my enormous thighs, wobbly arms and T-shaped belly button to my cankles, fat fingers and big toenails (some funny bastard once told me they looked like satellite dishes).

So how, then, with visible surgery scars across my back and under my armpit, a deflated left tit and a circle of back-skin where my nipple should be, had my self-confidence suddenly increased to the point of going topless before a herd of wild animals? Maybe it was because I was feeling better than I had done since my op. Maybe it was the antioxidant-tastic diet recommended by Smiley Surgeon. Or maybe it was my last hurrah before chemo did its worst. Whatever the reason, as steam came off the hair I was straightening the life out of, I wished I had the chance to go back to my thirteen/fourteen/fifteen-year-old self, give her a good shake and tell her not to be so bloody self-conscious.

'Anyway,' I said to P as I pulled on a posh frock for our dinner that evening, 'you ought to be making the most of my *hair*, not my body. In two days' time, mister, you're going to have yourself a short-haired wife.'

P leaned forward on the bed, brushing aside the sport section of his paper. 'Well, can my long-haired wife get over here, then, so I can make the most of her before dinner?'

Every website and leaflet and message board I'd exhaustively pored over since my diagnosis had recommended that the best thing to do before chemo was to cut your hair short. They said it would make the hair loss less traumatic if I didn't have to wake up to long strands on my pillow, and apparently it'd make me feel as though I was 'regaining control'. But, on the morning of my cut, as I cried at my reflection while straightening my shoulder-blade-length hair for the last time, in control was the last thing I was feeling.

My super-supportive (even for the seemingly ridiculous hair stuff) friend Tills had planned the perfect Chemo Cut day: an antioxidant-filled lunch, the haircut and then a spot of shopping to buy something to suit my new style. On the cab ride into town, I studied every passing woman's haircut – just as I had done with their boobs before my mastectomy. Who could carry off what style? Was it the long-haired or the short-haired women who got the most male attention? (Neither, as it goes – but apparently hot-pants can do a lot to help.)

Tills saw me through the window as I pulled up outside the café. A nanosecond's glance at my face told her all she needed to know, but rather than pander to my nerves, she set to pointing out sexy, short styles in magazines and telling me how fabulous I'd look.

The lure of a glass of champagne was the only thing that got me over the threshold of the swanky-yet-intimidating salon at which she'd booked the appointment, but when it became clear that their head stylist instinctively knew what would suit me (and recognised that I was as nervous as Pete Doherty in a customs bust), the whole experience became more fun than fearful. My best-ever hairdressers experience, in fact.

To save me from full-on scary shortness, the hairdresser recommended a compromise of a graduated bob that was short and funky yet feminine and, frankly, fabulous. So fabulous, in fact, that I hurriedly emailed a bunch of my mates, asking them to join me in a pub the following night – a sneaky ploy to (a) take my mind off chemo the following day and (b) ensure they saw me looking my best before the chemo drugs rode roughshod over my appearance.

As part of my diversionary tactics in the meantime, I arranged to meet P outside our favourite local restaurant that night. Sitting on a bench outside – not our usual spot – to sip a spritzer in the sun, I watched as he walked down the hill towards me, completely oblivious that it was his wife outside the restaurant. He even reached out to open the front door, then turned left to double-take the girl beside him. 'Oof!' he exclaimed enthusiastically. 'Wow, you look so young!'

'Shall I take that as a compliment, then?'

'Yes! Hell, yes,' said P, getting a better look by tilting my head with his hand on my chin. 'But bloody hell, I'm not half going to look old beside you.'

'Not to worry, love. I'm not half going to look bald beside you.'

'Oh shut up,' he said, shooting me a disapproving sideways glance.

'Shut up' seemed to be everybody's answer to my hair-loss gags. Not least the group of friends I met in the pub the following night. I found myself back in full-on compere mode – as I had been in the hospital after my mastectomy – being impossibly smiley, making wisecracks, giving the people what they wanted. 'Get me while you can, folks,' I said, wafting a hand past my new hair as though I were in a shampoo advert. 'By the time this little lot's fallen out, I'm never going out again.'

The new barnet went down pretty well with my mates. And by 'pretty well', I mean that I walked out of the pub with an ego the size of Texas. And by 'walked' I mean stumbled – my two-glass limit was more than enough to see me tipsy. (Apparently, chemo nerves + minimal alcohol = bumbling idiot.) I drunkenly waxed lyrical to P all the way home about what brilliant mates I've got, how I wanted my normal life back as soon as possible so I could carry on pissing about in pubs with them, how fortunate I was to be going through The Bullshit with such an amazing support network (sheesh, I must have been drunk – I said 'support network'), and how, despite The Bullshit, I still considered myself the luckiest lass in the world. It might have sounded more impressive and heartfelt had I not followed it up with a range of comedy accents.

Speaking of which, there was a terrific sketch-show moment that night. There we were, sitting around a table, talking about my boobs (as you do) when a charity collector walked over, shaking her tin. 'Money for breast cancer, anyone?' I'm sure the last thing the poor lass was expecting was for twelve people to laugh in her face, spitting out beer in hilarity, so we were understandably met with a stern, breast-cancer-is-no-laughing-matter look. We explained our reasons for finding her request so funny, but she obviously took that as a further piss-take.

'But you *look* all right,' she said, peering at me accusingly over the rim of her glasses.

'I might now, love,' I said, pushing a folded fiver into her tin. 'But come back and see me in two months' time, and I'll bet you the contents of that tin that I look pretty bloody far from all right by then.'

CHAPTER 10

The shape I'm in

So what does chemo feel like? To quote my spot-on chemo nurse, it's completely different for everybody: like childbirth, no two experiences are the same. Want to know what chemo feels like for me?

The first night after having the chemo drugs was horrific. I was a mug for thinking I could bring some cheery charm to the proceedings by glamming up for the hospital last week, flouncing into the Gloomiest Room In The World in my floral skirt and tottering heels like a lost shopper who'd been sent to Primark instead of Prada. Because, within hours of leaving the hospital, the not-so-floral reality hit me. Can't-keep-anything-down sickness, shakes and shivers, diarrhoea, wanting to rip out my veins, fainting, aching, heart palpitations, all-over bone pain, sweating, panicking, total inability to process my own thoughts, watching as my joints swelled and my skin developed itchy rashes, being able to do nothing but sway and say 'for fuck's sake, for fuck's sake, for fuck's sake' over and over. Can you imagine how difficult that must have been for P and my parents to witness? (My poor folks have not only had to live with the fact that their daughter has cancer, but that she says 'fuck' a lot.)

The days thereafter, while 100 per cent better in comparison, have still been cripplingly challenging. Nausea, exhaustion, aching bones, headaches, stomach pains and – worst of all – a complete messing with your head. Chemo (at least the first night after having it) must be like heroin addiction or cold turkey: it mucks up your looks and screws with your mind. It turns you into a different person. It takes away who you are and makes you 24/7 tearful and depressed and confused and paranoid and tetchy and unable to understand anyone around you. It makes you irritable and annoyed with the people closest to you, when all you want to do is tell them that you love them *so* much, and that they're the only reason you can be arsed to go through all this, and that without them there'd be no point.

How do so many people do this? Just how have so many people managed it and seen the other side? I'm only a couple of days into my first cycle and already wondering how I can spend the rest of the year handling this shit. For probably the first time since this all began, I'm feeling really bloody blood-boilingly angry and hard done by. I am twenty-fucking-eight. On the hottest weekend of the year, I should be sitting outside a pub in the glorious sun, drinking lager shandies and talking to my man or my folks or my mates about where to go on holiday, who's doing what for New Year, whether there'll be a series three of *Gavin & Stacey*, or what Derby County's chances are for next season. Instead I'm craving a cold, dark room, a few hours' decent sleep and a way out of this physical and mental . . . I don't know what . . . unfairness. Going through chemo has got to be the pinnacle of human endurance.

There's not a lot more I can say. Chemotherapy is a motherfucker.

*

That post came three days after my first chemo. And those seventy-two hours in the meantime were among the most miserable of my life. It had started well enough – dressing up for my first appointment, painting on as good a brave face as Max Factor could manage, doing my darndest to swallow the painful tears that threatened to fall in front of my husband on the way to the hospital, and smiling in the face of the strange looks I got upon entering the chemo floor.

As P gripped my hand tightly in the waiting room, the first thing that occurred to us was just how much hanging around there was going to be. First, you're weighed and measured. Then there's a blood test to check your white-blood-cell levels. Then the wait to find out whether those levels are okay. Then an even longer wait while the chemotherapy drugs are prepared. We could have flown to Spain and back by the time my treatment began.

But before all of that was a consultation with my oncologist – the same Glamorous Assistant I'd seen the week previous. 'Good news,' she said as we sat ourselves down in her office. 'Your CT scan came back clear.'

'Omigod,' I blurted. 'You're sure?'

'As sure as we can be,' she said. (It wasn't quite the triumphant 'absofuckinglutely' I was after, but it was good enough.)

'That's really . . . that's just . . . it's completely . . .'

'Amazing,' said P, finishing my sentence for me. 'It's amazing.'

'So we really know what we're up against now,' said Glamorous Assistant. 'As you know, the scan can't pick up the smaller cancer cells, but they are precisely what your chemotherapy is designed to treat.'

Harshing my mellow somewhat, she then reread the list

of possible side effects I'd heard the last time I'd seen her and I nodded along with each one, optimistically assuming that, at worst, I'd only be affected by a portion of her list. Because, really, how bad could it be?

While eating our M&S lunch of couscous and salad on a bench near the hospital, I received the call to say that my chemo was ready, and P and I headed back, our fingers still locked, to the second-floor room where my treatment was about to begin. I chose a seat in the corner and P pulled up a stool alongside me, giving me that pursed-lip, you're-being-so-brave look without actually using the B-word I'd recently banned. While getting hooked up to my cannula, being suspiciously stared at like a giraffe in a monkey enclosure by the other fifty- and sixty-something women, I asked my nurse to give me a hint about which of my two chemo trios I could expect to be the worst.

'Heck, darlin', it's just so different for everyone,' said the first, beckoning over two other nurses to get their opinions. One thought the first type would be worse on a sickness front, but that the second would be more painful for my body. The other said neither was 'a picnic', but that most people found the second type tougher to handle because of the accelerated hair loss. Then the first nurse waded back in, interrupting another chemo patient in the middle of her Maeve Binchy to get her take on the debate. 'Pff,' she exclaimed, looking over the top of her book and shrugging in a way that suggested I couldn't possibly understand at this early stage, before returning to the page she'd left. The nurses looked back hopefully to see whether my fellow patient's exhalation had answered my question.

'Righto,' I said. 'Better get on with it, then.'

Before being wired up to the drugs themselves, I first spent an hour with my head in a freezer. Or, at least, it felt that way. I'd read the occasional success story about cold caps – designed to cool the scalp, thus restricting the chemotherapy drugs' access to your hair follicles – and had begged on a previous visit to be given use of one. I'd have done anything – *anything* – to increase my chances of clinging onto my lovely locks and, catching sight of my cold-capped reflection in my iPhone screen, I realised just what that 'anything' entailed. I looked like a prize twat. 'This had better fucking work,' I spat at P from beneath the uncomfortable weight of my pink, coastguard-chic head-gear, and he did his best to hide his sniggers behind the back page of the paper.

Persisting with the cold cap meant a longer stay at the hospital, since its best chance of working was to wear it for an hour before and after – as well as during – the administering of the drugs. Which, in total, was a good five hours' worth of looking like an idiot. Not that the drugs themselves did anything to help. The steroid came first and, despite being the one that sounded like it would do the least damage, it immediately made me feel as though someone had put itching powder in my knickers. What is it with these drugs and their insistence on messing with your nether regions? There I sat, blushing beneath my freezing twat-hat, scratching my bits like a thrush gold medallist. So much for being the most glamorous girl in chemo.

'Tell me that's the lot of it,' I said to the nurse before she produced a bag of scary-looking fluid. She shook her head. 'Sorry, darlin', but it's time for the good stuff.'

The first batch of the good stuff was red – bright red, in fact, like a thicker version of Tizer. 'Now don't be alarmed,' said the nurse as she set it off on its journey into my veins, 'but your wee will be this colour later on.'

I pulled a face. 'Well, that'll be interesting,' I replied.

'And this red drug is the one that's mostly responsible for any hair loss,' she continued, flicking my IV.

'Or not,' I said hopefully, raising my eyebrows towards the cold cap. 'I'd better not be wearing this sodding thing for nothing.'

Once the first bag had found its way into my body, it was time for the second – this time a clear fluid that didn't look any different to a saline drip. The red stuff had looked like it might be painful but, in fact, wasn't at all. The clear drip, however, had a stranger effect. I felt hot around the throat and more than a little woozy. The third bag of drugs – also clear – wasn't much better, making me feel partly like I was underwater and partly fizzy in my nose, as though I'd eaten a whole pack of Haribo Tangfastics in one sitting. P and I tried to take our minds off the obvious by challenging each other to a water-drinking race (in the hope that it'd flush the red liquid through my system) and watching episodes of *Gavin & Stacey* on my iPod, but time passed slowly. I replied to all the texts I'd been receiving, wrote a blog post and did some work from my chair. P read a newsagent's worth of tabloids and continually kept my folks posted on my progress as they made their way from Derby to London, to be there in time for our return from the hospital.

Scooped-out jacket potatoes with cheese and bacon were waiting for us when we got home; Mum's caring, comfort-food method of healing.

'So how do you feel, Mrs?' asked Dad, and I didn't know how to reply.

'Dunno. Weird. Like something's about to happen.' And I wasn't wrong. Because, in the time it took to publish the blog post I'd written at the hospital and eat half a jacket potato, I'd taken to my bed, feeling dizzy, queasy, shaky and completely bloody terrified. I didn't know what was happening to my body, nor did my body know what was going on either. Even before things got to the horrible depths I wrote about in the blog post at the beginning of this chapter (the post that *still* evokes that bleach-like hospital smell and a sickness in my stomach), there was an overwhelming sense in my body that whatever had been put into it had to get out – and as quickly as possible. Hence the Lisa-shaped hole in the wall connecting my bedroom to the bathroom.

'Whose is that?' I said, pointing to the silver washing-up bowl on my bedroom floor as I climbed back into bed.

'I bought it,' said Mum, 'in case you needed it. To save you running to the bathroom.'

And then, right on cue – even before my head had touched the pillow – I jerked bolt upright, grabbing the bowl to regurgitate the couscous I'd had for lunch. Suffice to say, I haven't eaten couscous since.

When you're sick on a hangover, a relief usually comes from having barfed. But when you're sick after chemo – much like after food poisoning – you simply can't barf enough. As soon as Mum had emptied the plastic bowl, I'd need to use it again and, thanks to a carefully placed mirror opposite the bed, I could see that I was getting greyer with every puke. One moment I'd be sweating, the next shivering. My heart raced so fast that it made me panic, then the panicking made me faint, and the fainting made me delirious. I couldn't focus, I could feel my joints swelling, and I became convinced that my nose was growing too big for my face. I felt like I'd been poisoned. And, I suppose, I had.

I knew how ill I was. But if I had been in any doubt, all I had to do was look at the faces of Mum, Dad and P – they were petrified. They took it in turns to sit with me; Dad curling up beside me to hold my shaking hand, Mum bringing me ice cubes to suck when I couldn't keep down water, P mopping my brow with a wet flannel. 'Do you want the telly on?' they'd ask. 'Do you want to listen to some music?' 'Do you want a window open?' 'Do you want us to stay here, or do you want to be alone?' But the truth was, I didn't know what I wanted. I wanted nothing. I wanted to fall asleep, bypass the rest of chemo's immediate ills, and wake up when the agony was over.

What became clear after even the very first cycle of chemo was that, for the foreseeable future, I would have no significant concept of time. I'd sleep only sporadically, and at unusual hours. I'd eat only occasionally, and only once the smell from everyone else's meals had disappeared. Not even the promise of a *Coronation Street* double-bill could get me to the TV at my usual routine time. It was a miserable thing, made more miserable by the fact that the worst of it began on a Friday night and lasted all sodding weekend. I didn't even have the beauty of thinking, 'Well, at least everyone else is at work.'

By Monday, however, things had slowly begun to improve. Taking baby steps and holding on to Mum's arm, I walked to the nearest corner, and – more importantly – was finally able to enjoy a cup of tea. I was still super-exhausted, still felt a bit sick after as little as a minute of conversation, and everything still tasted like cardboard, but I was feeling more like myself and I wasn't half grateful. That's not to say that the effects of my first cycle of chemo had done their thing, mind you. There were still a few surprises to come. Not least the piles.

'Are you okay, love?' asked P from the other side of our locked bathroom door. 'You've been in there ages.'

'Fucking cancer,' I whinged from the loo seat. 'This sodding illness just gets more glamorous by the day, doesn't it?'

The hair loss, they tell you about. And the sickness, and the pain, and the depressing effect on your taste buds. But nobody warned me about the toll that cancer treatment was going to take on my arse. First the constipation, then the painful 'relief', then getting the runs . . . and then back to the start of the crappy cycle again. There on the toilet, squeezing my chest to my knees, I finally understood why, right back as early as my diagnosis, every cancer-experienced person I came across recommended that I keep a constant supply of Sudocrem. Bloody good advice – it's the single most brilliant gift you can buy a cancer patient. (Well, that and Louboutins.)

'P! Help!' I screeched from the loo seat, to the sound of hurried footsteps running down our hallway.

'I'm here, babe, what is it? Shall I come in?'

'God, no, don't come in,' I shot back in a single breath. (At this stage I was still fooling myself that I'd never allow P to see my bald head, so I'd have rather done an Elvis and popped my clogs there on the loo than have my husband see me as I was.) 'Just, erm, bring me something from the kitchen, will you?'

P's silence was deafeningly embarrassing.

'The olive oil, okay? Bring the olive oil.'

'Riiiight,' he said, scampering off to the cupboard.

'Don't look at me, okay?' I mumbled into my dressing gown while P held open the bedroom door for me after Sainsbury's best lubrication had done the trick. 'It's completely bloody humiliating.'

'Okay, beautiful,' said P – sensitive as ever – though I'd never felt further from beautiful. 'I'll leave you alone for a bit.'

Sitting on a travel neck pillow because I wasn't able to put any pressure on my damaged *derrière*, I figured things couldn't get much worse. But, looking up into the mirror opposite our bed to scowl at my reflection, I noticed that, in fact, it had.

'Oh, for fuck's sake,' I said, peering at the acne-ridden mess before me. Equally as startling as the nineteen spots I counted was just how quickly they'd appeared. 'Great,' I said, squeezing a zit on the end of my nose. 'That's just great. Because the puking and shitting wasn't quite enough. Now I'm getting uglier by the day.'

'Sort it out, scientists,' I wrote on my blog. 'What the hell is keeping you? You can send tourists to space, you can clone sheep . . . hell, you can make Posh Spice's tits stand up like *that* (thanks, Isaac Newton, your work here is done). So tell me, boffins, whose idea was it exactly to skip past the Making Chemo Bearable module and instead goof around growing human ears on the backs of mice? Or is this some sort of reverse-*Weird Science* experiment to create a hideous troll of a woman who'll actually consider getting off with one of you geeks? Because, well done, it looks like it's working. Get your lab coat. You've pulled.'

CHAPTER 11

Getting wiggy with it

August 2008

As cancer experiences go, I'm not convinced I'll have one quite as memorable as my first wig fitting. I'm rather entertained by the fact that I keep calling it a wig 'fitting', actually. That makes it sound like buying a wedding dress, when actually the two experiences couldn't be more different. In one, your mum cries while you spend an hour trying on a frock you'll wear for twelve hours. In the other, you cry with laughter while you spend fifteen minutes trying on a wig that you might have to wear for twelve months. The only similarity is showing off in front of a mirror although, again, in one experience your reflection looks as good as it ever will, and in the other your're staring back at Rod Stewart.

On the NHS, you're entitled to an acrylic wig, paying a prescription fee of about £60 (human-hair wigs bought privately can cost anything upwards of £1,000). It was never really my intention to go down the acrylic route, but I figured I'd take what I'm entitled to and see how I get on with it. Plus there's a tiny, foolishly optimistic part of me that thinks that since I've not lost any hair yet, it might just hang on in there, and that I'll never need a wig. Probably the same part of my brain that thought they'd got it wrong about the breast cancer. If needs be, though, I'm perfectly prepared to throw some money at the problem (the Louboutins can wait) and buy myself a real hair wig from a specialist shop, but for now I'd rather not have to think about it.

The NHS being the NHS, there was zero sense of style in the process. Instead, P and I were ushered into a hospital back room the size of a stationery cupboard by a disapproving little man with surprisingly small feet. The stationery cupboard had very high shelves displaying mannequin heads with truly awful hairdos that Wig Man had to stand on a chair to reach. (Wig Man is, by the way, completely bald – I wonder if he tries on the wigs when nobody's looking?) The lower shelves were home to an ancient-looking radio buried among lots of boxes containing wigs that had been ordered for other patients. I had a sneaky look and noticed that most of them were grey – another reminder of the lottery-winning odds of getting The Bullshit at my age.

Wig Man handed me a catalogue and told me to point out the styles that appealed to me most. I was tempted to show him a curly black wig reminiscent of The Scousers, but I feared this wasn't a man to be joking with. (Which, of course, made it even more impossible for P and me to stifle our laughter when 'Getting Jiggy With It' came on the radio.) I pointed out a couple of bobs and one or two longer styles to give him an idea of what I would be after, and he pulled down a handful of wigs from the top shelf, sat me in front of the mirror and combed back my hair so it wouldn't show beneath the wigs I was trying on.

Oddly, Wig Man referred to each wig as though it were an actual person ('She's too square for you, try this – her style is much more suited to your face shape'), but then I guess a little craziness is permitted when you spend your life in a hospital cupboard listening to Crap FM with only mannequin heads for company. Anyway, after quickly realising that the longer wigs made me look a bit like the lead singer from The Darkness, I tried a bob with a parting and fringe a bit like my usual hair, only fuller. And, to be fair, I was pleasantly surprised at how natural it (sorry, *she*) felt for an acrylic wig. But – let's be frank, here – I was still staring back at me in a wig.

Once you've chosen your design, you fiddle about with swatches until you've found the colour that most resembles your own, then go back in again once your order has arrived. If you like it (sorry, I mean *her*) you hand over your £60, then take your wig to a hairdresser who'll hopefully be able to cut it into a style that's a bit more contemporary. I'm hoping that, when I finally settle on a wig I like (and, let's be honest, I'm not going to find it on the NHS) I can persuade a fabulous Covent Garden hairdresser to style it, so I can avoid going to some dreadful wig-cutting-for-the-over-fifties place called 'Hair To Stay' or 'Curl Up & Dye'.

*

It started with the pubes.

And, in cancer's trademark spoilsport fashion, it happened on an otherwise glorious day. Finally able to be left on my own after the first batch of chemo, I was basking in the emancipation of feeling even slightly better after having been so ill. (Just to clarify, feeling good when you're having cancer treatment is different to the normal feeling good. You're not up for the usual nights in the pub, you don't look so hot and you get pretty knackered after, well, most things. But none of that makes it any less brilliant.)

So I took my chirpy self out for a walk up the road to buy

a Frappuccino, wearing my look-at-me Mickey Mouse-emblazoned hoodie. Even walking along my street felt better than it ever had. There I was, walking to the local café like a normal person, having seen off Chemo 1 and looking ahead to the next cycle knowing exactly what was in store. I must have looked like the local crazy, thinking about it. Your average Londoner isn't that comfortable with the sight of a wonky-boobed, grinning idiot with a spring in her step, as one woman demonstrated by looking me up and down in horror as we passed on the street. 'What you don't realise, love,' I thought to myself, 'is that the fool you've just walked past is actually an amazing woman.' Then I quickly chastised myself for being so damn cocky and empowered. Apparently cancer was turning me into Germaine Greer.

The shitty thing about cancer (not the only shitty thing, obviously, but it's pretty shitty nonetheless) is that it'll sneak up on you and piss all over your chips the precise moment you think you're finally in control of it. And so, later that same day, I found myself lying in bed with an embarrassingly musical arse and nagging constipation pains (a problem resolved by breaking the World Prune Eating record), and wondering just how long it would be before I felt sexy again. And then I went to the toilet and (cue chip-pissing) looked down to discover that a handful of pubes had come out on the loo roll.

'Shit,' I exclaimed, startled at the discovery. 'And so it begins.'

I had read that pubes are often the first hairs to go and, in all truth, their falling out was hardly an unwelcome side-effect. It was just what the pube-shedding symbolised: next, it would be the hair on my head. I dragged myself back to bed and told P the news. 'Why do these things have to happen?' I whinged, and promptly burst into tears. And, to my surprise, so did he.

It might have been my hair there on the Andrex, but that didn't mean that cancer's uninvited consequences were only having an impact on one person. Because once again I was reminded that this wasn't just happening to me; it was happening to *us*. P may not have been wired up to the drugs or experiencing the side-effects or seeing his pubes come out in clumps, but it was clear that he was feeling every bit of it. Arguably more so, thanks to the added frustration of being forced to play spectator, unable to do a single sodding thing about it. Having to watch the person you love go through that kind of stuff must be a horrible, helpless position to be in. But being married to a man who not only understood The Bullshit but felt it all too and, better still, didn't treat me any differently because of it was a pretty special thing.

It's an unusual position to find yourself in, lurching between Major Cancer Event and vapid nothingness. It's like lying on your back in a field, trying to catch sight of a shooting star – for ages, it's agonisingly dull, but then along comes a dazzling streak of light and then there you are again, without a schedule, waiting around for who knows how long. And that's another of the shitty things about cancer (expect to read that sentence a lot): just how utterly boring it can get. As small mercies go, at least my tumour had the good sense to show up in time for Wimbledon, a summer of cricket, the Olympics and the start of the football season.

On one otherwise dull weekday while P and Dad watched golf on TV, I stood eating lemon curd from the jar and staring out of the kitchen window, worrying that, with so little going on, I'd never again have anything interesting to blog about. I found myself willing something to happen – and there's the fatal error. Because, when I went into the bedroom to change out of my hooded sweater, I pulled it over my head and with it came a clump of my hair.

Despite my optimistic hope that my hair would stick around, deep down I guess I always knew that this day would come. But that doesn't mean it came as any less of a shock. Cue hysterical crying. P and Dad ran in to see what was up – how lucky that two of my favourite boys were around to give me a cuddle (Dad) and instinctively prise the hair from my hands and flush it down the loo (P). The tears continued for a long time, but once I'd got over the shock, I realised that it wasn't so much the hair loss I was crying about, but more the fact that I could have been so bloody cretinous to think there might be a chance – however small – of getting away with it; of this not happening to me. I hate being wrong at the best of times, but that dumb denial really took the cake.

So there it was. The hair loss had begun. And while it wasn't a horribly massive – or even noticeable – clump of hair that came out, it was still enough to know for certain that this was the beginning of the part I had feared most. Declaring my head out of bounds to anyone around me, I was overly cautious for the remainder of the week, desperate to retain as much hair as possible before my next chemo session. No longer would I rub my hair with a towel, or comb through conditioner in the bath. Where I'd usually have washed it most days, now I was letting my hair go without its usual application of shampoo. To my mind, greasy locks were infinitely preferable to a Bobby Charlton comb-over.

But even comb-overs need washing occasionally and so, three days before my second chemo, I gave it a go. I ran a bath, lit a few candles, put on some chirpy tunes and set to it. I stuck to all the cancer hair-care rules (super-gentle massaging, pH-balanced shampoo, lukewarm water). I even allowed myself to think for a second that I'd got away with it. But when it came to the drying (low temperature, slow speed, wide-tooth comb, yadda yadda), that was where it all unravelled. Literally.

Even when drying without the necessary combing (if I'd have left my hair to dry on its own I'd have ended up looking like Gene Wilder, and that's worse than bald), hairs were flying right off my head. Run a comb through it, and they were coming out even easier. Foolish as it may now seem, I carried on drying and combing as little as I could get away with, figuring that for as long as I had hair, I wanted it to look as good as it could. But still it thinned and thinned, covering my back, my shoulders, the floor, the bedspread and filling the baggy left cup of my bra. It was e-v-e-r-y-w-h-e-r-e.

Imagining P's reaction to our new bedroom carpet, I set about scooping it up and, despite having watched as it all fell out, I couldn't get over the amount I collected. In fact, I was so surprised by it, that I saved the shotput-sized hairball and put it on the bathroom window-sill so I could later show it to P. Just a couple of days previous I could get away with running a comb through my hair. Now, I could barely stand in a breeze.

To my surprise, I didn't cry. I sat and stared blankly at myself in the mirror for a good twenty minutes, testing out headbands to disguise my thinning locks. But when, later that afternoon, I spoke to Dad while I drove into town for an afternoon at work, and he made some minor comment about my hands-free kit and questioned my ability to hear other cars on the road, I totally lost it.

You know those stupid, niggling worries that you sit on for a while, then in the heat of the moment they pour out of your mouth all at once, at breakneck, Vicky Pollard speed? It usually kicks off with the words, 'And another thing . . .' (or, 'Yeah but, no but . . .'). Well, that's exactly what happened. What I should have said to Dad was that he and Mum had been incredible from day one, that no one could have done more for me than they had, and that I couldn't imagine how difficult it must be for them to watch their daughter go through this . . . but could they perhaps remember that while The Bullshit may have been having many effects on me, it hadn't robbed me of my ability to drive, my ability to make good decisions, or my ability to look after myself in the way my doctors had advised.

But, of course, it didn't come out like that. It was more along the lines of: 'For crying out loud, Dad, just because I've got cancer doesn't mean I'm incapable of driving, you know! And you need to realise that [sniff] I'm not a little girl any more and [snort] I'm doing all the right things and [splutter] the symptoms are [whimper] not. my. fault. The acne's not caused by fizzy drinks and the piles aren't down to my sodding diet [sob] – they're because of the BLOODY TOXIC CHEMICALS in me [snivel] and it's time you fucking trusted me to look after myself!'

Dad told me that I was right, that he was sorry, that he trusted me and that parental instinct sometimes made him and Mum say the wrong thing. And, of course, that made me feel even worse. Those things needed to be said (maybe not in the way they came out), but saying them didn't make me feel any better. Because nobody deserved to be on the end of my criticism less than my Dad. My folks aren't just parents. They're my best friends. And, as much as I might sometimes want to tell them to do things differently, I should instead have shut my trap for once and showed gratitude for the millions of things they'd done so brilliantly.

None of us knew the right way to handle The Bullshit. Cancer doesn't come with a manual. Every symptom and every emotion feels so different for each bloody unlucky sod who's forced to live with the shitty disease, so who knows the best way to play it? As for me, I could handle the surgery and the chemo and the illness and the hair loss. But difficult conversations with my family? That was where I drew the line. Let's just call it the hair that broke the cancer patient's back.

CHAPTER 12

Back in 'therapy

I keep forgetting how dangerous this disease is. It's something I've been doing all along, even straight after hearing the words, 'signs consistent with breast cancer'. My immediate reaction wasn't 'shit, that's life threatening', but 'bollocks, my hair'. Even in chemo last week, when a number of doctors warned me to keep my arm still for fear of the drugs seeping out of my veins and into my skin, causing massive problems, I still couldn't help but gesture wildly and continually reach inside my bag to show the nurses my iPhone/magazines/photos/lip gloss.

I actually think that conveniently ignoring the scary stuff is a damn good tactic. It ensures you never frighten yourself by thinking too far ahead, and forces you to deal with the more pressing business of just putting one foot in front of the other. That wartime 'keep calm and carry on' slogan is a design for life, if ever I heard one. (But try reminding me of that after Chemo 2 tomorrow when I'm puking and panicking, and I'll bite your ear off.)

While staying in Derby with my folks over the last couple of days (P's been away with work on a team-building excursion – three words that give me the willies as much as 'breast cancer'

– I've caught up with lots of different people who I've not seen since my diagnosis. And, while lovely, their reactions to me have been another reminder that other people seem to be more terrified by The Bullshit than I am. Not that they've been overly sympathetic, weepy or pitying – quite the opposite, thankfully. There are a lot of things I want (free iTunes downloads and an hour in a locked room with Dave Grohl for starters) but pity is categorically not one of them. So instead of commiseratory head-tilting, everyone has instead offered giant, beaming smiles that scream out how pleased they are to see me.

It's brilliant to be on the receiving end of that kind of reaction (and also makes you feel a bit like a celebrity). I've had hugs and kisses, been picked up and squeezed, had heartfelt arm-rubs and meaningful back-slaps. When I saw my eighty-six-year-old uncle, his eyes (and mine) filled with delighted tears as he gave me the loveliest cuddle and said, 'I've been trying so hard to think what you'd look like, but it's you! It's still you!' And he, by the way, has got more than enough to occupy his mind right now, let alone what I look like. His wife, and my amazing auntie, is also in the middle of cancer treatment, and yet is still as magnificent and matriarchal as ever. As she made me a brew, showed off her new wig and gave me a lesson in syrup-shopping, my uncle leaned over to me and said, 'You know what? I still fancy her more than ever.' Here's hoping P says the same when Chemo 2 sees off the rest of my lovely locks tomorrow.

*

'Are these presents?' asked the girl behind the counter in Accessorize, as I handed over £100 worth of headscarves and headbands that I wouldn't have ordinarily looked twice at.

'Nope. They're all for me,' I replied, choosing to spare her my cancer tale and instead allow her to assume that I was some kind of hair-accessory fanatic.

'There ought to be a grant for this stuff,' I whinged to P as we walked back to the hospital, where my chemo drugs would be waiting for me.

It was emergency headwear shopping – that morning, another chunk of my barnet had ended up down the loo, resulting in a nice, obvious bald patch right in the middle of my parting – and I resented the expenditure. The following week, I was going to have to fritter a fortnight's worth of mortgage payments on wigs. Granted, I'd spent twenty-eight years wasting my money on stuff that would barely see me through a season, but that was *my* choice. Having to splash the cash out of cancer-dictated necessity was just plain unfair. (I have issues with Clearblue for precisely the same reason. Hundreds of pounds' worth of pregnancy tests, ovulation sticks and digital thermometers, and still no baby? I should have just made like Madonna, saved myself the hassle and bought one on eBay.)

I had been in Sarcastic Sod mode for much of the day, not helped by the fact that I got sat next to Holy Mary while having my cannula put in. There was so much hanging around and staring at other people in chemo that, having been twice, I'd had the chance to size everyone up. Along with Holy Mary, there was Wonky Wig, Glamazon (pink slingbacks and blingy jewellery), French Stick (skinny Parisienne), Head Honcho (fabulous headscarves) and Speaking Clock, who I adored, despite the fact that she barely came up for breath. (I suspected I was known as Get A Room, on account of the glued-to-my-face husband.)

It was very stiff-upper-lip in the chemo room; everyone quietly waited their turn and smiled politely, with no dramatics or serious conversation. Until Holy Mary rolled up, that is. That day, she was having a go at her nurse for not having baptised her children. 'If they die, they'll end up in purgatory!' she shrieked at a volume that wasn't entirely appropriate for a room in which some of the patients' days were so obviously numbered.

Sensing the poor nurse's inability to find a suitable answer, I butted in. 'Well, there's a happy conversation for the chemo room to hear,' I chirped, as my Irish nurse fiddled with my cannula and – with perfect comedy timing – shouted, 'I can't get this little fucker in!'

Even Speaking Clock was lost for words, and gave me a cheeky wink as we watched a stunned Holy Mary turn more Holy Ghost as her horrified face drained of colour.

Having a giggle with the nurses from beneath my twat-hat (foolishly, I stuck with it in the hope of clinging on to my remaining locks) made the hours pass that bit faster, and the extra attention I got from them – a seat by the window, extra cups of tea, Fox's Glacier Mints – suggested that I'd gained a few popularity points as a result. But the fun had to stop sooner or later, and within half an hour of getting back home – too soon, even, to enjoy Mum's comfort food – I was, as Dad would say, 'singing into the big white telephone'.

Later, as I puked into the silver plastic bowl that now made me retch when I saw it, I realised I'd learned nothing from the couscous episode – this time, I'd scoffed a cheese baguette at lunchtime, and the results weren't much better. In fact, so rank was the smell (not to mention taste) of my cheesy regurgitation that I had Mum take away my bowl, despite not being finished with it. So much for the pristine, white pyjamas that she had so lovingly washed and ironed.

You have to be careful what you eat pre-chemo. If I'd

carried on that way, treating myself to foods I loved on an otherwise grim day, I'd have had nothing left on my Favourite Foods list. But even that was changing by the day, making way for the only things I could stomach at a time when even tea and toast looked as appetising as a dog-turd kebab.

I was fast developing other favourites – my chemo survival kit, if you will. Marmite was right at the top (and, Marmite haters, don't knock it until you've been through chemo); the one thing I fancied in chemo days one to three. Ice cubes, too. The relief of an ice cube dripping water onto your tongue when you've been barfing all evening and your mouth feels like the inside of a hamster cage can't be beaten. And then there was ginger. Ah, lovely ginger. Ginger biscuits, ginger tea, ginger sweets, crystallised ginger . . . I even had ginger bath foam.

Not that knowing how best to survive made Chemo 2 any easier than #1. Though I definitely managed the physical stuff better the second time around. During the first cycle, I couldn't believe that it was possible to feel that lousy and come out the other side. But, of course, you do. And that meant less panicking the second time around. (If not less swearing. Some things will never change.) What it didn't mean, however, was less of the mind-messing, or less of the depression. Because Chemo 2 didn't just bring with it the same old side-effects as last time. This time it took my hair as well.

Suddenly, with hair falling out entirely of its own accord, the hairball on my bathroom window-sill seemed pathetic in comparison. And it wasn't even falling out evenly. Instead, it seemed to be coming mostly off the crown, leaving me with a balding patch on the top of my head and longer strands still holding their own at the sides – think

Andy from *Little Britain*, or Keith from The Prodigy. Now I wasn't just a cancer patient – I *looked* like a cancer patient. And now, the wig-shopping wasn't just a game – it was a *necessity*.

As hard as I tried to turn it into a joke, there was a horrible truth beneath the humour. Because, if I was going to stick to my guns of being as honest as possible about my breast cancer experience – to my family and blog readers alike – I was going to have to 'fess up about just how difficult it was becoming. 'This blog isn't a performance or a novel,' I wrote. 'It's my *life*. My real life. Hence this is doubtless an often frustrating, up-one-minute-down-the-next read. But that's got to be the way it is, because that's the way my life is.'

I hated admitting the depths I'd sunk to, but it was important that I did. And so I recounted on my blog the morning on which I woke up at 5 a.m. in floods of tears.

'What's wrong, angel? Was it a bad dream?' said P, rolling over to give me a cuddle.

'No. I woke up,' I replied. 'And I didn't want to.' I was livid with the world for allowing me to wake up, and for putting me through cancer's shitty ways for another miserable day. As much as it disgusts me to admit it, at 5 a.m. that day, I'd rather have packed it all in.

I'm ashamed that I woke up feeling like that. Because that's not how I think. It's not how I do things; it's just not me. Kissing me on my bald patch, P held my tearful face in his hands. 'I never want to hear that from you again,' he said. 'Because if there's no you, there's no me either.'

'I'm sorry, darling,' I said, 'But—'

'But nothing,' P interrupted, now crying himself. 'Nobody said this was going to be easy. But you've got to do it. You've *got* to. I *need* you to.'

We both knew that some days were going to be like this. Some days I just wasn't going to have enough energy to feel like I could keep going. And, as difficult as that was at the time, for me and everyone around me, sometimes, it was just going to have to be that way. 'Difficult' doesn't do it justice, of course. This wasn't difficult. It was near fucking impossible. Because, when the shock of the diagnosis goes away and all the initial attention you get dies right down, what are you left with? A big, ugly, horrible, grim, morbid mess to scrap your way through, and nobody can fight it but you.

But I'd do it. Of course I'd bloody do it. And despite the lows I'd been feeling, I didn't mean it any less. What choice did I have? This awful, awful thing came along, and it changed the course of my lovely life – of *our* lovely lives. We didn't ask for it, we hadn't planned for it, we'd done nothing to deserve it. We HATED it. But I loved my life more than I loathed that cancer. And I was going to get it back.

CHAPTER 13

Does my bum look big in this?

As I type, I'm looking down from my bed at a foreign, furry, blonde rodent, otherwise known as my new wig. It's balanced carefully on a stand on the floor and, despite the low light in here, it still looks glossy and healthy and wholesome. It's everything I'm not.

Next week it's my birthday, and the one thing I wanted was to still have fabulous hair by that point. (I wanted a gift-wrapped Dave Grohl too, but apparently you can't always get what you want.) Next best on the birthday wish-list, then, was to have a fabulous, non-NHS wig. Ta-dah! Today, I got exactly what I asked for. And I hate it.

There's nothing wrong with the wig I bought today. It's a damn good wig – as good a wig as I'm going to get, that's for sure. It's just that the whole wig-buying experience was so . . . oh, I don't know. Don't get me wrong, it was a whole lot better than the stationery-cupboard NHS experience. Wig Man was replaced by Wig Girl who had a far better understanding of what would suit me and how it should be worn. And this time, I didn't just have the moral support of P, but also my wonderful friend Tills. Even by the time P and I arrived, Tills had got the

106

measure of Wig Girl and the designs she had to offer, and had even picked out the mops that would suit me most. Everything was in its right place, going as well as it could. But this time it was real, and not just pissing about in front of a mirror with Crap FM on the radio. (Actually, that's a bit of a fib – apparently, all wig places listen to Crap FM.)

Trying my best to be a cool customer and perfectly at ease, I slapped on my brave face and even played along with a few of the usual losing-your-hair lines. 'Just think of all the money I'll save on highlights!' and 'Blimey, P, I'll be able to get ready so quickly!' Ha ha ha! Well, no, actually. Not ha ha. Because, I realised, this is fucking rubbish. Here I am, at twenty-eight, trying on wigs. Not for fun, but because I've got breast cancer. Not so funny now, eh? And it was about that point at which I lost my sense of humour, got really bloody angry and burst into tears.

I quickly asked Tills to tell me about something else that was happening in the world. She recalled a story about our friends' little girl, who recently threw a tantrum when her mum gave her a biscuit, and nobody could understand why. Much questioning revealed that the issue with the biscuit was that it was slightly broken, so it was quickly replaced with another one from the same pack. But that brought on an even bigger tantrum because, in fact, what the (frankly, genius) little lass wanted was the very first biscuit she was handed, just without the broken bit. She wanted the perfect version of her original biscuit. Just like I wanted the perfect version of my original hair. I was having the same tantrum.

In my tantrum, though, I sobbed and had a go at two of my favourite people for telling me how great I looked, when what we were really looking at was a cancer patient in a wig. 'The reason I've got you two here,' I spluttered, 'is not so you can tell me what you think I want to hear. Stop fucking telling me I look good. I look like I'm wearing a wig.'

In these angry, shouting-at-people-I-love moments, what I want is someone to really kick the crap out of. But, because I'm lucky enough to only ever be surrounded by lovely people, there's never anyone to kick the crap out of. So instead, my most incredible, supportive, wonderful friend gets it in the neck, after giving up her morning to be with me for this ridiculous wig-buying charade. I don't just want to do all this crap-kicking because I got breast cancer in the first place, or because I feel so ill or because I've lost my hair. I want to do it in retaliation for turning my time with Tills from cava-drinking, tapas-eating loveliness into shitty, cancer-focused experiences like this.

I know those times will come back. And then some. But I really miss my mates, dammit. I'm sick of being the cancer patient on the sofa, talking about myself and skirting around the truth of how very, very shit all of this is, in case people don't want to hear it. I want my mates to see me in normal circumstances with a brew, a load of gossip and a bloody lovely head of hair. I want them to say, 'Wow, Lisa, I honestly can't believe it's a wig! It's exactly like your old hair!' And I want them to mean it. But again, that's one more thing I can't have. Because if anyone does say that, they're lying.

*

'I know, I know, you were expecting the wig,' I said, greeting my boss, Kath, at my front door.

'So where is it, then?' she asked, peering suspiciously at the LA Dodgers baseball cap that made me look like even more of a fruitcake when coupled with White Company pyjamas.

'On the bathroom window-sill. And it's staying there. I fucking hate it.'

'I'll be the judge of that,' she said, dropping a bag of goodies on the nearest chair and marching down the hallway.

'That's it? It's nice!'

'Yeah? You try wearing it.'

'And the headband . . .?' questioned Kath, upon looking a little closer and finding the rug styled up with an Alice band.

'Oh, that. I'm just trying it out. Seeing what I can do to make it look more like real hair.'

'But it *does* look like real hair.'

'Mm. Until you put it on your head,' I concluded.

After all the support she'd given me, the least I could have done was let Kath be the audience to my wig's debut performance. I felt bad about it – I should have given her a glimpse of the bald head by way of compensation. People want the good stuff, right? And that was the weird thing about my reluctance with the rug. People knew I'd had a mastectomy; I was happy to show them the scars. They knew I was having chemo; I was happy to show them the baldness, and yet I still wouldn't let them see me in a wig. And so I'd spent £200 for the privilege of displaying a syrup on a stand. This was getting ridiculous.

There was nothing wrong with the wig in particular. For short periods at least, it didn't feel all that unusual to wear. And, admittedly, it looked better on my head than it did on the stand. But it still didn't look like my old hair – and it was never going to. Like it or not, I had to get used to it, and so I set a new rule: if I couldn't have my own hair, then I was damn well going to have everyone else's. This was simply Wig 1 of a New Wig Army. I wanted a shelf of wigs like my shelf of shoes. I wanted a wig for weddings, a wig for work, a wig for shopping, a wig for the pub. I was going to be a wig slag. Apparently I just wasn't a love-the-wig-you're-with kind of girl.

I don't know why I expected to love the wig immediately. In fact, I've always been rather suspicious of anything – and anyone, for that matter – that instantly impresses me. I'm a big believer in the slow burn. Even when I first met P, I hated him. I took his initial shyness as arrogance (I believe I told a colleague he was 'practising to be a git') and did all I could to avoid him around the office. Which just goes to show that first impressions often mean squat. And, true to form, the same seemed to be happening on the wig front.

My intentions of wig-slaggery seemed to be paying off: from hating the sight of Wig 1, within a matter of days, I had come to actually quite like it – and its new sister, Wig 2. The wigs, by the way, came with names. Not names I had given them, you understand. (An ex-boss once told me about a brilliant naming system he and his wife devised to covertly ensure her wig looked good when they were out at a restaurant. 'Have you seen Sharon recently?' she'd ask. 'Is she well?' To which he'd reply either, 'Oh yes, she's fine,' or 'Well, I think she could do with a lift.' Genius.) The thing is, all wigs have names already – names to distinguish them from one another in the catalogue and, my God, how brilliant they are. Wig 1's name was Codi. Wig 2 was called Erika. (I wonder whether people switch from jobs in paint-naming to wig-naming?)

I bought Wig 2 (sorry, Erika), from a different Wig Place to Codi. This time, it wasn't Wig Man or Wig Girl, but Camp-as-Christmas Wig Guy – the best of all the Wig Folk so far. He was ace: the perfect mix of a damn good laugh, super-knowledgeable and understanding of the reason I was there in the first place. He even offered to shave what was left on my head to make the wigs fit better. I politely declined, opting to GI Jane it in my own time. (The following morning, as it happened – so much hair came out in the bath that P and I nonchalantly took the scissors to the lot of it, making me less Andy-from-*Little-Britain*, more Aryan army recruit. Call it Hitler Youth Chic.)

Camp-as-Christmas Wig Guy stuck rigidly to the wigs' catalogue names throughout my appointment. 'Samantha's lovely; see the way she's feathered around the face. Let's try her and let's take in Miranda too.' (Disappointingly, there was no Carrie or Charlotte.) And, despite thinking I'd walk out with a long wig, I found myself still unable to wear one that didn't make me look like a member of the Mexico '86 England squad. Thus, Wig 2 was another bob. A longer one, though, with a slightly wispier fringe. And this time it was Spring Honey, in comparison to Wig 1's Creamy Toffee (see what I mean about the paint-naming thing?).

My insatiable, hussy-like appetite for syrups even had me looking into Wig 3. In anticipation of my appointment at yet another Wig Place, I began looking at their wares online, and was so excited by the daft names that I set to sharing the joy on an email round-robin with my mates. Because, at this place, the wigs didn't just have women's names, they had brilliantly wanky titles like Emotion, Ecstasy and Rendezvous. There was even one called Ominous. But my favourite by far was from the Delboy Trotter school of wig-naming: Tres Bien. *Très Bien*! Now that, I thought, could definitely work in a covert restaurant wig-checking situation. '*C'est bon?*'

'*Tres Bien*, Rodney, *Tres Bien*.'

In the meantime, though, it was time to stop taking the piss out of the wig industry and get to the more pressing business of actually stepping out of the flat in one of the buggers. I'd spent years faffing with my hair, demanding impossibly high standards from it. (I'd better clarify that I'm talking post-schooldays, by the way – 1990–1995 was a half-decade hair-mare. With that and the braces, it's amazing I ever got a snog.) I'd blow-dried, straightened, sprayed, lacquered, highlighted, lowlighted . . . all in a quest for the perfect 'do. Newsreader hair, if you will. That pristine, shiny, well-conditioned, weather-proof, always-looking-perfect kind of hair that just doesn't exist. Or does it? Because, as it turned out, the perfect hairdo was achievable – but it wasn't without its drawbacks.

August bank holiday was Get Over Yourself And Show People The Wig weekend. And I think it's fair to say that it made an impressive debut. Sorry, *they* made an impressive debut. First up was Wig 2 (a choice I still don't understand, given that Wig 1 was always my favourite). My future sis-in-law Leanne's hen party was that weekend and, knowing that I wouldn't be able to stay the course for the Big Night Out, I instead showed my face for an hour at the pre-cocktails picnic. Well aware that twenty-something hens can be tough crowds, I had never felt more self-conscious. It didn't help that, as I tentatively walked towards the tiara-wearing group with my sunglasses perched on top of my head (because that look's got 'natural hair' written all over it, right?), I promptly got my Aviators stuck in my wig and had to prise them out in the middle of a busy Kensington Gardens. Suffice to say, I chose not to wear my designated hen-party tiara.

That's what I mean by drawbacks: leave your wig alone, and it's perfect; start to fiddle, and you've given the game away. The thing is, wigs are itchy. For about twenty minutes, they're surprisingly comfy. After that they're just plain irritating. And when I've got an itch I'll scratch it, which meant that my fringe suddenly had the ability to grow beyond my eyebrows in a matter of seconds, and my parting could magically move two inches to the right without the help of a comb. I might as well have left the label hanging out.

Everyone was very complimentary about it, though, even the unlikeliest of praise-givers – namely my mate Jon. Despite being one of the most thoughtful men you could hope to meet, Jon isn't one to offer up an easy compliment, even at a time when you might need it most. (I remember once going to meet him in town while we were seeing each other. I was trying really hard to look impressive despite a crippling hangover and I thought I'd done a decent job, too, until I strutted over and he said, 'Wow, you look like shit.') A couple of days after calling round to see me, he rang to give me his verdict. 'Now, there's something I've got to tell you,' he said, ominously. 'The other day when I was round at yours I was, of course, aware that you were wearing a wig. Because you've told me about it, and because I've been reading about it. But when I was sitting talking to you in your front room, I wasn't thinking, "Here I am having a brew with Lisa in a wig," but, "Here I am having a brew with Lisa." After initially seeing it, the wig just didn't occur to me at any other point.'

I appreciated Jon's ruling on the rug. But then, I guess, he was hardly going to go, 'Sheesh, Lis, that's one dodgy syrup you've got there.' But whether or not he was blowing smoke up my ass, it didn't matter. Because, for the meantime, when baldness was the only alternative, wearing a wig was as good a second best as I was going to find.

CHAPTER 14

My Super Sweet 29th

September 2008

There's something wrong with my tear ducts. I've been back through all my chemo leaflets and lists of side-effects, but it looks like this is one thing I can't blame on the drugs. The problem is me – I'm turning into a cry baby. Over the past week, I've felt happier than I have at any point throughout The Bullshit, and probably even happier than I've felt for a while before it. Last night I almost felt guilty for being so chuffed with my lot – cancer isn't supposed to feel this good, surely? So why do I keep sobbing at the slightest thing?

On Friday I cried in two different taxis (London cabbies, you have been warned). The first was on my way into the West End to head back to the office for the first time since my diagnosis. And wow, I'd almost forgotten I lived in London. Pretty much all I'm seeing of the city at the moment is the view from the car on my way to the hospital, but on Friday I looked up from the cab window and found myself on Westminster Bridge – Houses of Parliament on one side, London Eye on the other. It felt like I was seeing it all for the first time, and I beamed so much it brought tears to my eyes. The capital has never looked so beautiful.

Then I cried on the way back home, this time from a mix of emotions; most of them wonderful, some less so. But first, the wonderful. Being back in the office was weirdly exhilarating. Everything had a new excitement to it: the dodgy lift, my swivel chair, the banter, the tea in a chipped mug, the compliment on my top from the woman on the front desk, my stationery holder (I'm very fond of my stationery holder), flicking through schedules, being able to talk about something other than cancer . . . it was knackering, but fantastic. But best of all was being around people again. Not that I've been locked in a cage for the last couple of months. What I mean is being around people in a normal, everyday setting. I hadn't realised how much I'd missed it.

And then there's the less wonderful stuff. For every few people in the office who smiled and winked and said hello, there seemed to be another who completely ignored me. One even stared straight through me when I looked him in the eye and said 'hi'. I appreciate it's difficult for some people to know what to say, knowing what they now know about me. And I'm definitely not expecting people I don't know to suddenly start being all friendly because they feel they ought to. But being ignored by someone you'd normally talk to every day is a pretty shitty thing, and makes you feel a bit like a leper.

Then, after my cab ride back from the office, a similar thing happened – I arrived home at the same moment as my normally-very-chatty upstairs neighbour who, upon seeing me, couldn't get away fast enough, using a poorly improvised cold as her excuse (which didn't stop her going out for a jog later on).

Thankfully the people who matter still treat me exactly as they always did – actually, better than they always did, judging by this weekend's barrage of birthday love. Which, of course, had me crying even more – several times, actually. Reading cards, opening presents (not least the scouse wig I was bought, but that may have been for different reasons), during a show at the theatre, when my family and friends left my flat after a lovely afternoon cake-fest . . . you name it, I cried at it. All my talk of booze-free, tame celebrations might have been true, but it didn't make my twenty-ninth any less fantastic than any other birthday. In fact, I dare say it was better than my last few birthdays put together.

So why all the tears? Having spent most of today thinking about it (to the point where my brain hurts), I think the reasons are three-fold. (1) I'm overwhelmed. Since The Bullshit came along, my life has had to be a bit slower paced. So perhaps the emotion-packed excitement of the last few days was almost a bit too much to handle. (2) Tiredness. I'm like a baby at the moment – let me have the requisite sleep and food, and I'm a little angel. Allow me to get tired or hungry, and you'll wish I'd never been born. (3) Fear. All these wonderful things and all these wonderful people . . . it's something else, I tells ya. My life is the stuff that dreams are made of. And while I wouldn't change any of it for the world (apart from the obvious), every now and then it reminds me how utterly, completely, wake-up-in-the-night *terrified* I am that The Bullshit has come along to put it all in jeopardy. How fucking dare it.

*

Only when you've got cancer and it's your birthday is it acceptable for your friend's husband to buy you knickers. It's a little-known present-giving loophole that Tills' husband Si took advantage of when they handed over my birthday gifts. And they weren't just any old knickers, oh no. They were the Best Knickers In The World: a white thong with 'Mrs Dave Grohl' on the front. (P loves them, as you can imagine.)

The special treatment that had been threatening to wane post-diagnosis was suddenly back on my birthday, and a morning of call-taking, present-opening and bouquet-receiving left me exhausted. Tills suggested that a method of breast-cancer-payback would be to exploit people's kindness for all it was worth, and start blogging about how Miu Miu shoes and Chloé handbags would really aid my recovery. She was right, of course, but not about the exploiting bit – recent studies have conclusively proved that being bought designer gear is the quickest way to stave off cancer cells, and you can't argue with that.

It's a dreadful thing to admit, but I was kind of getting used to all the thoughtfulness I was being shown. Not that the people around me aren't normally kind to me, you understand (I think we've already established how fortunate I am on the friends-and-family front), but I feared that it was going to turn me into a horribly spoilt, me-me-me brat like one of those awful kids on MTV's *My Super Sweet 16*.

Earlier in my birthday week I had spent a gloriously happy afternoon giggling on the sofa and watching that very show with my brilliant friend Busby. It inspired us. During the course of the show we devised a plan to make my birthday next year, well, super sweet. Party-wise, my twenty-ninth birthday celebrations had to be a little on the tame side (theatre, restaurant, tea and cake), but then, what was so special about turning twenty-nine anyway? Thirty is the big one. And in the hope that, by the time I hit the big 3–0, I'd have a lot more to celebrate than just a new decade, Busby and I stayed true to our Virgoan selves by planning my shindig WELL in advance. With a little help from the pampered princesses on MTV.

'Right then,' said Busby, 'there are rules to adhere to if you're having a Super Sweet birthday party.'

'Do elaborate,' I replied, dunking my ginger biscuit in my sixth brew of the day.

'For starters, you're going to have to look like *that*,' she said, pointing at a house-sized teenager, bursting out of the seams of her hideous pink frock and whinging that she didn't think her parents would buy her the right car.

'Looks like my folks will need to remortgage their house to buy me a new Audi as well, then.'

'Only if it comes wrapped in a huge pink bow,' said Busby. 'And at some point, it seems, you'll need to have a massive strop at your mum.'

'After which she'll cancel my credit card and I'll call her a bitch in front of a shop full of people,' I concluded.

'Oh, and your dad—'

'You mean *Daddy*,' I corrected.

'Yes! *Daddy*. Well, he'll be responsible for booking a performer – and, obviously, anyone less than P Diddy would just be, like, totally lame,' continued Busby, now in an American accent. 'And you'll have to invite your school crush and give him access to the VIP area! But then he'll make out with another girl and you'll get security to throw her out.'

'And he'll come back grovelling when he catches sight of my super-fly Audi,' I added.

I missed this type of daft banter that comes from idle Saturdays on a sofa with your mates or Friday afternoons in the office. It wasn't that The Bullshit had put a stop to me acting up with the likes of Busby, but how much sweeter it would have been if I hadn't been wearing pyjamas and a wig. The cancer-centred grind of the past couple of months had been enough to make me forget how good all of this stuff could be.

Not that it's difficult for me to forget stuff at the best of times. I'm known among my family and friends for two things: always being late and having a terrible memory. I forget names and dates (an affliction I keep on top of with a ridiculously organised diary and a propensity to write lists), important tasks, whole conversations, nights out, childhood memories . . . you name it, I've forgotten it. I can barely remember anything I learned at school, college or uni. (Except to only use a colon after a complete statement. And never begin a sentence with 'and'. Oh.)

Oddly, the same amnesia applied to chemo. Despite having been through it twice, I still couldn't remember exactly what it was going to be like. So I was bricking it even more at the thought of Round Three, which was looming over me like an apocalyptic cloud.

CHAPTER 15

Old red eyes is back

In chemo on Friday, one of the nurses commented that I looked 'very glam'. If only she could see me now: I look like a smackhead. The first couple of days post-chemo went pretty much as I'd come to expect. My folks may have hit it on the head when likening that first night to watching someone in torture – they're now convinced that chemo drugs are used for that purpose, and I'm not going to disagree. Ask me what you like in the midst of those few hours and I'll tell you *anything* to make it stop.

Anyway, I'm through the worst of it again now. Not that it's made me feel any chirpier, mind. I'm three chemos down, which means I've got three to go. And while everyone keeps going on about how brilliant it is that I'm halfway through, what I can't believe is that I'm ONLY halfway through, dammit. And by being 'through the worst of it', what I mean is that I feel a tiny, tiny fraction better than I did a couple of days ago. I don't feel as sick now, I've stopped hallucinating (this time, as well as the now-standard feeling that my feet and hands are expanding, I was convinced I had a lump growing beneath my left nostril), and I'm definitely standing up straighter whenever I have to move anywhere (not that the being-accompanied-to-the-loo days have passed yet; I'm hoping that's a treat I can look forward to tomorrow – that and a nice, private number two once my course of constipation-inducing pills is over).

But boy, they're right about the tiredness symptoms being accumulative. I feel like a frail old woman. P ran me a lovely bath yesterday with posh Molton Brown bubbles and candles all around the tub, but all I found myself craving was one of those old-person baths with a door in the side that fills up around you and saves you collapsing on your husband when you climb out of it. Sheesh, it's a good job we live in a ground-floor flat, or I'd be scouring the ads in the Sunday supplements for a Stannah stairlift too.

The best thing about getting past the first four days, though, is not having to sink a handful of pills every few hours. The steroids do their job (if 'doing their job' is not only to make me feel less sick, but to gain weight at a speed that would impress Mr Creosote), but they end up starving you of any decent sleep at a time when you've never needed it more. For me, that means lying awake and thinking about things that I wouldn't normally consider. Like getting a tattoo, for instance.

A few days ago, I received a referral letter to see the radio-therapy department about the course of pain-in-the-arse sunburn (actually, make that pain-in-the-arm-and-tit sunburn) that I'll be starting in December once the chemo is done with. And along with the letter came an information sheet telling me what radiotherapy is all about. It all seemed pretty standard – daily visits for six or so weeks, lying on a computer-operated bed, burned skin, feeling tired, yadda yadda – but there was one thing I hadn't bargained for: the tattoos. Now there's a thing I hadn't realised you could get on the NHS.

Apparently, they give you three small tattoos (dark blue dots) to ensure the radiotherapy is beamed at exactly the same area each time, and to guarantee they don't administer rays to the same place again in future, should The Bullshit come back. Granted, I'm hardly set to become the Amy Winehouse of breast cancer, but even so, I'm miffed. Because if I've got to have a tattoo, don't you think I should be getting them out of choice, rather than stupid cancer-dictated necessity?

So, despite the fact that I've barely considered having one before, I've now started thinking I might get one done to celebrate getting through my treatment. Now's probably not the time to be making these kind of decisions, but who knows, perhaps after I'm through with The Bullshit, I might go mental and get a topless girl drawn onto my upper arm. Or join up the blue dots into a pocket-style tattoo, à la Winehouse. Because if The Bullshit is ballsy enough to make a recurrence in the future, the radiographers can damn well work around my new body art. And, for the record, if it ever does come back again, I'm going all out and having 'oh for fuck's sake' tattooed across my forehead. Once round The Bullshit is more than enough, ta very much.

*

As an addition to the lovely Jo Malone treats he'd bought me for my birthday, P also handed me a tiny parcel. 'It's just something daft,' he explained. 'But I want this to become your new mantra.'

I tore off the wrapping, and pulled out a fridge magnet upon which was a Winston Churchill quote: *Never, never, never give up*.

'Promise me?' asked P.

'I promise, babe,' I said. 'Of course I promise.'

It was a promise that Dad reminded me of the morning after my third chemo.

'I need you to do something for me,' he said, curled up beside me as I lay in bed, a shivering, dejected mess ravaged by the treatment that was supposedly making me better. 'I need you to take the advice on the fridge magnet that P got you. I know how difficult this is for you right now . . .'

'No you don't,' I shot back.

'You're right, shitface. I don't.' (Even in chemo's most miserable moments, Dad and I would still refer to each other with our usual, less-than-flattering terms of endearment.) 'But you've come this far, Lis, and we're all so proud of you for doing it. Just please – *please* – promise me you'll keep on going.'

'Oh-kay, doofus,' I mumbled reluctantly.

Being halfway through my schedule of chemotherapy brought with it its own issues: on the one hand, everybody's congratulations on how far I'd come allowed my mind to wander to what might happen afterwards, and how I might celebrate when The Bullshit was done (the getting-a-tattoo plan had not gone down all that well with my nearest and dearest). But on the other, being three chemos in meant that I was all too familiar with the drill – and the regular hospital trips were starting to piss me off as much as the treatment itself.

I'd begin each Chemo Friday by picking a fight with P out of sheer tantrum-inducing frustration. Yelling at him had become my coping strategy:

'You're seriously wearing *that* T-shirt?'

'What do you mean you're going to buy a paper? You're supposed to talk to *me*, not gen up on the US Open.'

'I left that light on for a *reason* – now just fucking leave everything alone, will you?'

'Look, are you walking two steps behind me or *with* me?'

This time, I even stormed out of the flat and attempted to hail a taxi on the street, despite our minicab being scheduled to arrive a mere ten minutes later. It was mean and it was irrational, but it was my reaction to having to turn up to an appointment that I knew would later make me feel – and look – like death. By the time we'd reached the hospital, I'd have wiped away my tears, reapplied my mascara and apologised to P. I wanted him to see me the way the chemo nurses saw me – cheery and fearless and impossibly lovely, not some tetchy bitch who shouts at her husband.

P told me recently that it was all he could do not to snap back at me in those moments, and that he was as frustrated as I was that he was having to force me to get into a one-way cab to hell. He hated not being able to do more to help, which was probably why, as soon as I was able to get back out of bed again after each round of chemo, he went into helpful-husband overdrive.

With my taste buds as obliterated as my hair, we had figured out that it took around four days for me to be able to taste anything. Everything between Chemo Friday and Tuesday tasted like carpet. Cancer leaflets tend to liken taste to cardboard, but I always found that lacking a bit, since food in those first few post-chemo days actually tastes of nothing. Not cardboard. Not even carpet. Just nothing. Whatever I was eating might have tasted like wax or feet or concrete or fabric softener for all I knew.

Being the chef around these parts, P devised Fajita Tuesday – his method of finally doing something con-structive. For two chemos running, it had proved a sizzling success. And despite the fact that not even my favourite lunch (a cheese-and-crisps sandwich and a mug of tea, simpleton that I am) had hit the flavour-spot earlier on in the day, I was becoming impatient to get my favourite sense back with P's chilli remedy. But this time, nothing doing.

'Doing the trick, love?' he asked, expectant hope glistening in his eyes.

'Mm-hmm,' I replied, keen not to ruffle the chef's feathers. (Even on a normal day, if P gets a verdict of anything less than 'absolutely delicious' for the meal he's cooked, he's in a strop for the rest of the night.)

'I put loads of spice into this one, you see, but I didn't want it to blow your head off.'

'No, no, not at all, babe – it's just the ticket,' I said, pushing peppers around on my plate and nodding my head a little too vigorously.

P put down his fork. He meant business. 'It's not working, is it?'

I said nothing.

'It's not bloody working. You can't even get any joy from fucking food any more, can you? Stupid. Sodding. Bastard. Cancer.'

The Bullshit's screwing with my scran was the last straw for P. He's not just the head chef in our household, but a bloody brilliant one to boot. P takes his cooking *very* seriously and, like every successful chef, he's a competitive little bugger. And he wasn't going to be beaten to the palate punch by my chemo drugs. So he picked up our plates, stormed back into the kitchen, emptied the fridge of vegetables and started waving a huge knife around like Crocodile Dundee at a blade-throwing class.

'I'm going in for the kill,' he shouted back to the living room. 'And this one's going to work.' I kept out of the way for as long as I could hear expletives, and sheepishly headed in an hour or two later to find a huge pan of super-spicy, master-blaster, chock-full-of-chilli soup on the stove.

125

'Leave that there overnight,' he said, when I enquired whether I'd be expected to see off the lot there and then. 'By tomorrow, that little baby's going to sort you out.'

And, by heck, it did.

Feeling calmer the following afternoon once my tongue's usual functions had returned, we headed back to the hospital for our first visit to the radiotherapy department. 'The reason we're doing this radiotherapy,' said Chelsea Consultant (very west-London posh in her Tod's loafers and a diamond engagement ring that could take your eye out), 'is that we want to localise the zapping of the cancer cells to the specific area where the tumour was, unlike chemotherapy which works on the cells all over your body.' All fair enough, I thought. And then came the bombshell. 'We'll be aiming the radiotherapy at not just your chest wall, but also your left arm and shoulder, and the left side of your neck. And the reason we're doing this over such a large area is to increase your chance of survival.' And there it was. Another cruel reminder of the grim, makes-you-want-to-scream seriousness of breast cancer.

It suddenly made the illness and the hair loss and the fajita-eating seem like welcome distractions from the fact that, actually, this thing had the potential to kill me. I *hated* having to think about that. I can't begin to describe how much of my flagging energy I used *not* thinking about that, always finding other things to occupy my mind (how do you think the blog came about?). So it came as a horrible, jolting shock when P and I *did* hear it. It wasn't that we'd forgotten that I had breast cancer in the first place (hell, I don't think a minute will *ever* go by in which I forget that I had breast cancer); it was that we had got so used to it being in our lives that the shock of being forced to reconsider its gravity was a little too much to bear.

The tattooed dots were going to be a ball-ache. But it was the reason behind having them that terrified me. I decided to look online to find out more about the process from other radiotherapy-experienced people. I'd kept out of online cancer-communities thus far, choosing instead to go it my way and save confusing myself with pages and pages of information that might not be relevant to me. I'd love to take credit for that decision but, in truth, it was Always-Right Breast Nurse's idea. All that mattered, she said, was dealing with my own experience, and that she or anyone else at the hospital would be able to answer any medical questions I had. And, true to form, she was spot on.

I quickly found a picture of someone's radiotherapy tattoos (I was pleased to discover they looked more like navy freckles than medical marks – not that it dampened my resolve to get a design of my own), and then I found myself engrossed in some message boards. But it wasn't the medical information I found online that left me confused – it was some of the comments in the chatrooms. Whether or not I was looking for it, I don't know, but I kept finding the following sentence: 'Getting cancer was the best thing that ever happened to me.'

Now I'm the first to trot out the 'each to their own' line but, to my mind, saying that kind of thing was completely fucking irresponsible. Granted, I hadn't seen out the whole of my cancer ride yet – and who knows how I was going to feel at the end of it – but I was pretty damn sure I wasn't going to thank my lucky stars for having been blessed with The Bullshit. Beckoning in P to read the words staring back from my laptop screen, he angrily confirmed that I wasn't alone in my opinion.

I could see the reasons behind people saying it. If their experience of cancer had been anything like mine so far, they too would have had the wonderful, *Amélie*-like moments where you're on the receiving end of so much love that the world seems a rosier place. And while all of that definitely helped, it didn't for a second mean that getting breast cancer was the best thing to ever happen to me. Because for every rose-tinted moment come a lifetime's share of dark times that leave you lonely and frightened and confused.

In a blind rage, I took to my blog. I didn't want anyone to think that getting cancer had been the best thing to ever happen to me, or that it could be the best thing to happen to anyone else, for that matter. It changes your life. It changes your outlook. And it changes *you*. But that doesn't make it a great thing. Cancer changes your life because it threatens it. Cancer changes your outlook because it muddies it. And cancer changes *you* in far more ways than just losing a boob or going bald or getting dots tattooed on your chest. Cancer IS NOT the best thing that could ever happen to you. Cancer, I'm afraid to say, is shit. And I was only part way through it.

CHAPTER 16

I'll be there for you

There's every chance you'll disagree with me, but I find the concept of 'best friends' a dangerous one. For kids it's perfectly acceptable, but when you grow up it's far healthier to have a group of mates with no person in particular being at the pinnacle. So why, then, have I suddenly started playing favourites with my friends?

It's not like I've got a Santa-style list of who's been naughty and nice, or even that any of my friends are aware of this behaviour (at least they weren't until now, but I'm hoping they'll let it slide on account of the cancer stuff – yes, that old chestnut). It's just that with me getting so much attention and support and wonderful gestures and love from so many of them, it's no wonder that they've moved up several places in my mates' league. Having done a bit of research (read: discussed it with Mum), it seems a lot of people view their friends in a core-of-the-earth kind of diagram, with their best pal(s) in the middle, their closest mates in a circle around that, good friends on the next layer, followed by see-less-often people and then acquaintances near the edge. But mine's become more of a hierarchy.

It's a top-heavy structure we have here at Friends Inc. (less pyramid, more ice-cream cone), and I'm a lucky CEO in that the top level of my hierarchy – director level, if you will – is jam-packed with magnificent mates. They keep me going: they're in constant contact, they make sure I'm up to speed on the world outside my cancer bubble, they don't treat me any differently, and yet they're happy to let me have a whinge if ever I need one. In short, they're brilliant, and they're all in for a serious pay rise once The Bullshit is over (i.e., the beers are on me).

But – cue more favouritism – within this level have emerged three friends (they know who they are) who really ought to have a level of their own. They've taken magnificence to new heights, this little lot, and if we were all still at school I'd form a special club for them and make membership cards and pin badges and devise a secret handshake.

Then there's the management level of friends – they also keep in regular contact, but probably not so much as the directors. They'll send the odd text and the occasional Facebook wall post, but they're always up to speed with my progress, love 'em, despite asking fewer questions than the directors (the blog helps a lot on that front).

Next is the shop floor. These small few are still in contact about as much as they ever were but, thus far, have made absolutely no mention of The Bullshit, despite being well aware of it. And that's fine (though it is a bit like me suddenly getting a bright green mohawk and them asking where I bought my shoes). In some ways even, I secretly appreciate it. Besides, at least the shop-floor few are still in touch, unlike the cleaning staff at Friends Inc.

The cleaning staff comprises a much, much smaller number of people who have suddenly stopped showing up for work and disappeared off the radar completely. I'm not just talking about a handful of 'mates' here, but mainly acquaintances who'd normally be in contact from time to time. 'Facebook friends', if you will – y'know, the ones who make up the numbers. Those same numbers that I suspect will suddenly dwindle as soon as I hit 'publish post'. (For the record, I'm not expecting folk to befriend me just because I've got cancer. That would make me the human version of Timmy from *South Park* and, thanks to the steroids, I suspect I'm more Cartman.)

Guilty fun as it may seem, I don't want to rank my friends in a Eurovision Song Contest-style league table, and I'm not daft enough to think that the world has stopped turning just because I've got breast cancer. Everyone's still out there, leading their normal lives, buying groceries, arguing about where to spend Christmas, shouting at referees, ironing holes in their shirts and elbowing space-hogging commuters on the District Line. It's a comforting thought, actually, so I'm hardly going to strike anyone who puts their regular routine in front of sending me an email off my Christmas-card list, ferchrissake. But that doesn't stop a mischievous part of me from wanting to update my Facebook status with: 'Lisa has still got breast cancer, in case you were wondering.'

*

I caused a bit of a stir with that post. ('I thought I'd better send an email this week before you relegate me to the cleaning staff,' said one mate. 'I'd better be at director level, lady, or I'll be handing in my notice,' said another.) And I was strangely pleased it had, because writing that post was cathartic – not just that, it also cleared up a few issues I'd hitherto been sitting on.

The fact that I was suddenly having to answer a hundred emails, though, was indicative of an obviously true chord I'd struck. There was no getting around it: while some friends had admirably stepped up to the mark (the over-whelming majority, actually), others were suddenly MIA. The best friends, however, were the ones who were still making themselves known even at this stage, three months past diagnosis when my cancer news had become fish-and-chip paper. And this, it turned out, was the time when I needed them most; the time at which I needed a big old push into my second phase of chemo.

Three months isn't a long time. If I'd fallen pregnant at the same time as discovering I had a tumour, for example, I'd have only just been getting around to telling people about it by now. And yet within that short time, cancer had done its dirty work – I was bald, bloated, boob-less and pretty bloody fed up about it. Everything had become so much of an effort – getting out of bed every day; trying to stay positive despite the obvious cancer concerns; convincing myself that every little twinge I felt and pain I endured wasn't a return of the cancer, but merely part of the treatment's effects.

One night I even convinced myself that an outbreak of blackheads signalled the growth of a new tumour. I had been warned to expect this kind of paranoia – and if I told you it had since waned, I'd be lying – but even I could see that worrying that blackheads = cancer was bordering on the ludicrous. But I still managed to whip myself into such a panicked frenzy that P had to physically lift me away from the mirror and put me in bed with tight sheets tucked around me like a mental patient.

I found it equally difficult not to look at myself in mirrors, especially since my flat is covered with them. But one evening before bed, while changing into my pyjamas, I caught sight of my mutilated boob and balding head in the mirror, and my ugly reflection hit me like a demolition ball. While I allowed myself the occasional sob about it, I worked hard at not getting too bogged down with fretting about my appearance, since there wasn't a damn thing I could do about it. But that night I really let it bother me, and ranted to P about how unattractive, freakish and undesired I felt. What I hadn't bargained for was how hurt P was by my comment: I couldn't understand why he took it so personally. And so, in my grumpy tiredness, I got the hump about it and stormed off to hide under the duvet, slamming the bedroom door behind me and ignoring the one piece of marriage advice my dad offered us in his speech at our wedding: never go to bed on a bad word.

Dad was right, of course (I don't call him Yoda for nothing). Rather than discussing why P was upset, I instead got angrier and angrier as I lay alone in bed. 'Why the hell should it upset him?' I thought. 'I'm the one suffering here – he looks as handsome as ever while I'm busy being beaten with the ugly stick.' But of course it upset him, and not just because I didn't look like I used to. Let's just reverse the roles for a minute: if it had been me watching P go through this, it'd have been equally difficult for me to see him suffer from the physical effects as it would be to stand by, helpless, as he took such a massive hit to his confidence and self-esteem.

Cancer can be so isolating sometimes and at that moment I'd forgotten that I wasn't alone; that this was affecting other people too. Rowing with P was a harsh way to be reminded that it's better to be angry together while cuddling in bed than it is to be angry in separate rooms. And so, in the early hours, that's what we did. P told me how cross he was that The Bullshit was so impossible to reason with, and I told him how cross I was about it coming along at a time when I had the most to lose: the plans we had for our future, the twenty-something fun I was busy having, and the looks I'd never appreciated.

I was livid (I still am, as it goes) that my body had been ruined by this awful fucking disease, and I constantly worried about other people's reactions to it. My in-laws were due to arrive to stay with us for a few days (P and I gave my folks Chemo 4 off, thinking it was time they went a whole six weeks without having to hold a sick bowl for their daughter), and I was scared that they'd be horrified by the change since they last saw me: back in July, I was just one chemo in and still had all my hair. Man, were they in for a shock.

It's a shitty state of affairs, worrying about whether or not your appearance might upset people, and worse when you don't have the energy to do very much about it. I knew from my conversations with Smiley Surgeon that a common initial reaction to being told you have cancer is, 'What will it do to the way I look?' But you're encouraged not to think about it too much, and instead to concentrate on your treatment schedule, keeping free from infection and staying as mentally strong as you can. But isn't having confidence in the way you look part of that mental strength? There's no way to avoid thinking about what you look like when it's there in the mirror, staring you in the face every sodding day.

Which is why, of all the help I had been offered on various leaflets and websites from numerous cancer charities, I only really paid attention to one: the one that confronted the appearance issue. Everything else, I figured, I could find my own way through. But this? This I needed some help with. Not least with Jamie and Leanne's wedding just three weeks away. I needed someone to show me how I could make the best of what I had been left with, and send me back out into the world feeling confident and beautiful. And that's exactly what I got.

Look Good, Feel Better is designed to help women

manage the visible side effects of cancer treatment. Having been given some information on the charity by Always-Right Breast Nurse (who else?), I sucked up the tears and booked myself in for one of their workshops. Met at the door by a representative from the charity (who did a double-take that had 'but you're so young' written all over it), I was ushered into a small conference room with six other women, each of whom gave me the same look. Not surprising, considering I was the youngest there by a long chalk. (I almost felt a bit of a fraud, actually, like Marla Singer in *Fight Club*, pretending to be a cancer patient just to pick up a few make-up tips. Thankfully the wig and a brilliantly timed hot flush gave me away.)

We each took a seat around a conference table and were given a sizeable bag full of make-up and skin-care goodies – all donated by the beauty industry – with different products to suit our skin tones, after which we were taught all the tricks that would fool strangers into thinking we were normal, healthy women. Looking after your skin at its most sensitive, drawing on eyebrows when yours have done a bunk, evening out your skin tone and covering up the blotchy red bits, making your eyes stand out when you haven't got eyelashes to rely on, hiding the dark circles . . . all the seemingly surface-skimming things that women with cancer really want to know but often feel daft asking about, considering the weight of the 'serious stuff' we were supposed to be focusing on. And yes, beneath the slap and the wig was the same old self-conscious me that cried at the sight of her body in the mirror. But knowing that it was possible to work a bit of make-up magic to make myself feel even temporarily terrific was worth its weight in gold eye-shadow.

CHAPTER 17

I shall be released

October 2008

Well, this is weird. My legs don't work too well, the signals from my brain are much slower in getting to my body parts, my heart is thumping, my bones are painful, I've got a dodgy tummy, I've been put on more than double my usual amount of bloat-inducing steroids (alas, it looks like it *will* be George Dawes doing a reading at Jamie's wedding) and I've got a weird taste in my mouth that's like sucking on coins. But I can't remember the last time I felt this happy.

Drumroll please . . . I've not thrown up! I still feel like complete shit, but at least it's a different kind of shit, thanks to my new type of chemo. Apparently a change *is* as good as a rest. From the moment Chemo 4 began making its way through my drip and into my veins, it felt totally different. I felt sicker sooner. But rather than it getting worse within an hour of me reaching my sofa, it instead began to ease, and the sick feeling sank from my mouth to my stomach, where I'm happy for it to stay. It even allowed me a crackerbreads-and-soft-cheese interval. And even the hallucinations gave me a break long enough to watch *The*

Goonies and *Sex and The City*. I did have a weird delirium in the night, though, where it felt like my teeth and tongue were growing too big for my mouth – but still, it was only the one, and this time it came without that pain-in-the-arse voice in my head. (It was always an older version of my voice I heard, annoyingly trying to coach me through the worst and give me ill-founded advice on what to do, like an embarrassing parent on the sidelines of a Sunday League football game.)

Actually, the whole process of chemo yesterday was better than it has ever been. Dare I say it was almost fun? Granted, Chemo Friday started as it usually would (this time I inflicted the crying fit on my in-laws), though P avoided the usual coping-strategy bollocking thanks to me directing my anger at the loo roll instead. It was doing that bloody irritating new-loo-roll trick where the layers separate and it only comes off in ripped chunks. I like my toilet paper neatly perforated, dammit, so I made it known by throwing the roll across the bathroom and watching as it landed in a wet-feet patch outside the shower. Which made me even angrier, of course, because I then had to do the pre-wipe, knees-together walk to the other side of the room to fetch it.

But from the moment we left the flat, everything went well. We had a smoother ride to the hospital by choosing to go in our own car, rather than suffering the questionable driving of the World's Dodgiest Cab Firm. When we got there, the receptionist gave us a Golden Ticket in the form of a free parking pass, thanks to my ongoing treatment (see, cancer's not without its upsides). I also decided to overdress for the occasion, beginning my new life-tactic of saving nothing for best. And I went prepared by uploading series two of *Gavin & Stacey* onto the iPod.

Things were even pretty fun in the chemo room itself. All the coolest nurses were on shift, including my favourite who swears as much as I do. There was a real Friday Feeling, too – it was quieter in there than usual, which meant more banter between the nurses, good sweets out on the counter, a bit of flirting when the male doctors came in and a whiff of gossip in the air.

And so, ill and old and wobbly on my feet and slow in the typing department as I feel at the moment, I'm also pretty excited. Actually, excited doesn't even nearly cover it. I'm emancipated. I know I may be speaking too soon (fave nurse warned me that the 'buggery bit' of this kind of chemo may come between days three and nine), but even the possibility that I may never again have to endure Puke Friday (at least, not of chemo's doing) is the best news I've had in ages. Knowing I've got all three cycles of that first f-u-c-k-i-n-g h-o-r-r-i-b-l-e chemo type out of the way is, I reckon, as close to the undoubtedly wonderful feeling of being told you're cancer-free as I can get right now. For the first time since The Bullshit began I feel that *I'm* back in charge. I can handle this. I'm on top of it. I've pulled one back. Is the worst of it over?

*

Stupid, stupid girl. Had I not learned that the Spoilsport God of Cancer would be reading that post? Within three days of assuming that the non-sickness of Chemo 4 made it an obvious improvement on the three that had preceded it, along came the gift of a brand-new menu of side-effects – excruciating bone pain, headaches, earache, loss of balance, thrush (both vaginal and oral, as a special treat), pins and needles and that same old impenetrable fog of depression.

I'd had enough. *Everything* was pissing me off, from the state of my tongue to the squirrels in the back garden and even people's well-wishes. I was an idiot for saying that the aftermath of Chemo 4 had been any better than the last –

not just in the statement itself, but in the resulting contact it elicited from delighted friends and family. They'd make calls and write emails and send messages to say how pleased they were that things were looking up – and all just in time for the 'buggery bit' that my nurse had warned me about. I wanted to strangle each and every one of them, but I barely had the energy to think it, let alone do it.

Whether it was out of sympathy or intimidation, people would continually tell me that having cancer entitled me to a whinge whenever I wanted one. So I found myself taking advantage of their kindness and cranking up the moano-meter at every opportunity. So much, in fact, that I soon became sick of it myself. In fact, I was bored of it all. Bored of whinging, bored of the side-effects, bored of the enforced sitting around . . . bored of cancer. The novelty had well and truly worn off.

As much as I'd probably have taken a vicious swipe at anyone who tried it, what I secretly wanted was for some-one to finally have enough of it, kick me up the arse and say, 'Oh, for fuck's sake, stop your whining, will you?' My mate Leaks did once courteously include me on a group email about a pub meet-up, despite knowing full well that I couldn't make it. 'Who's in?' she asked, to which I replied, 'I can't – I'm washing my hair.' She fired an email straight back: 'You're not still trotting out that old cancer excuse, are you?' And I loved her for it.

The thing was, despite The Bullshit having been part of my life for months, I still *could not believe* that I had cancer. You'd think that all the boob-and-hair-loss fun would have made damn sure the reality had sunk in, but no. It was just such a fucking ridiculous idea: me with breast cancer. Yeah, right! I wanted to laugh, it seemed so ludicrous. I was still half expecting to find out that it was all some kind of huge,

Truman Show-style experiment that Channel 4 were secretly filming. And no amount of me actually saying the word 'cancer' was making the truth any more believable. And it really should have, considering the fact that I said it all the sodding time.

It still came as a shock to hear other people say 'cancer' with reference to me. Shortly after the 'buggery bit' hit, in yet another of my pathetic, long-faced, sympathy-seeking moments, P pulled a blanket over me as I lay on the sofa, and I looked up at him with those pity-me eyes (that even *I* was annoyed by) and whinged, 'P, I'm pooooorly.'

'Well yes, of course you're poorly,' said P, with the patience of a saint on death row. 'That's because you've got cancer.'

I almost slapped him. 'What's he talking about?' I thought, before remembering that it was, in fact, the case.

Not everyone was comfortable saying the word 'cancer'. Even the nurses in chemo tried not to say it out loud, instead calling it 'it' or purposely missing it out of sentences altogether. ('Yeah, it's different with each day in here. All the women here today have got breast. Mondays is ovarian. And on Thursdays everyone's prostate.') One day I even caught Mum mouthing the word 'cancer' mid-sentence, in that over-enunciated, speaking-through-glass way that some people still revert to when saying 'lesbian' or 'black'.

But being able to say it aloud like Harry Potter says 'Voldemort' didn't mean I was any better equipped at handling it. This should have been a joyous, exciting time – Jamie's wedding was just days away, but not only was I unable to fully enjoy the anticipation of the happiest day of his life as I would have ordinarily, but I felt increasingly guilty for trumping my family's matrimonial excitement with my stupid bloody illness.

With my chemo schedules timed around the big day, things had been planned so that I'd be feeling better and ready to party just in time for the nuptials. But, anxious as I was to get to that stage, with Chemo 4, the getting better was more of a struggle. It was the movement thing, mostly – with my bones aching to a point where I was convinced some of them must be broken, I was shuffling about like a geriatric Quasimodo. And, with little more than a week to go before I had to pull my huge hat, strapless dress and four-inch heels out of my wardrobe, I was convinced that, come the wedding, I'd look more Neanderthal than *Homo sapiens*.

Jamie's wedding was the only thing pulling me through my depressive lull. And depression was what it was. I had thought that all my whinging was just me taking the opportunity to have a moan, and letting the bubbling-under-the-surface anger have its moment but, as my procrastination became more painful, I had to concede that it was more than that. I was cross with myself for confessing it. I *hated* having to say it. Depression was a word I loathed. Like 'stress', I saw it as a term that was bandied about too much by people with no sense of its meaning. To my mind, telling people I was depressed made me look weaker than I liked to think I was. It was admitting defeat. But it was the truth.

In reality, depression is something that is stuck, rigidly, in your mind (or your soul or your body, I don't know), that shows its face only when you allow it. Not that you consciously allow it. It senses when you're vulnerable and lacking the compulsion to keep it hidden, and surprises you with a mini mental breakdown in the middle of *Deal or No Deal*. It makes it impossible to do all the little things that show the world you're okay: laughing at a joke, winking at your husband, tapping along to a tune, enjoying a cup of tea, idly singing to yourself as you get dressed. It presents you head-on with all the worries you try so hard not to think about: that the treatment's not working and you might be dying; whether you'll make it through the night; whether or not you can trust your family to pick a decent song to play at your funeral; whether you've got time left to listen to all the favourite albums you've not heard for ages . . . The worries get more and more ridiculous as they come, and it's the trivial ones that panic you the most.

And then, as the panic reaches its peak, it all implodes in your head and you're left with a bleak, grey nothingness and uncontrollable weeping that makes you tell your dad – the one person you most want to keep up the front for – that you've got no fight left in you and that you haven't got the energy to go on. And then you feel even worse for letting him hear it, and it leaves you not just with chapped, raw, painful eyes from all the crying, but a gut full of guilt from letting your favourite people in the world hear all the stuff you've tried so damned hard to keep from them. You go from a strong-on-the-outside, brave-faced girl to a consumed, cloaked, troubled mess with a dark side to rival Anakin.

All of it – all the blogging, all the banal things I talked about, every stupid sentence I said that didn't reveal what was underneath, every time I set the Sky+ for *Coronation Street*, every smile I'd offer and joke I'd crack and 'I'm fine' answer I'd give – ALL of it was a gargantuan effort I was making not to let the dark stuff surface. Because it was there all the time. Cancer forces you to act. And soon the acting becomes the reality, because you're so bloody determined to put out the right signals, come across a certain way and get the better of the stuff that could ruin it all for you. It was the role of my life: my Hannibal Lecter, my Don Corleone, my Scarlett O'Hara. And it was exhausting. But I was going to have to pull it out of the bag once more for the sake of my beloved brother. And I don't think I could have done it for anyone else.

CHAPTER 18

Pull out the stopper

Ooh, it's all go in here. Morning suits hanging from every curtain rail, hat boxes out in the spare room, marks on the carpet from new shoes being worn in, and me and Mum look like we've been dipped in gravy after getting a spray-tan. Oh, and a certain kid brother of mine is sitting beside me with a grin the size of a banana (let's see if he's still smiling at me tomorrow when he realises who fed his best man all those stories).

I'm equally smiley. Fancy me having a social life again, eh? I'm starting to forget what it was like to be out among people, acting daft and putting the world to rights over a G&T. The other night I spent longer than I care to admit trying to remember every detail about my favourite London pub, wondering whether they've cranked up the log fire yet, if the flush in the toilet on the left has been fixed, and whether the colder weather has forced my drinking buddies to move from the benches outside to the rickety stools in the bar. Classic withdrawal symptoms, I imagine. But I just can't shake the feeling that I'm being left out of a brilliant social scene and loads of gossip and good times that I'll never be able to catch up on.

Those very same drinking buddies met up at the pub in question on Friday night and, by heck, was I narked. My mate Lil sensed as much and, the moment she got back home, updated her Facebook status with: 'Lil had a great time at the pub but really missed Mac.' Much as I appreciated Lil's efforts to make me feel better, I'd had a whole evening of sofa-bound boredom to work myself up by then. I knew full well how ridiculous it was to get so wound up, and tried to console myself with thoughts that my mates weren't, in fact, having a blinding time without me but had instead been plotting to make and sell charity T-shirts with 'Save Mac' on them, and debating which bands they could get to play at Mac Aid. But of course they bloody weren't. They were drinking dodgy wine, slagging off *X Factor* contestants for their transparently insincere tears (I'm telling you, I could sob my way to the final of that thing next year) and eating endless bags of crisps, the carefree gits. It's not like I think the world should stop turning just because I've got breast cancer. But the least everyone could do is put their social lives on hold until I'm better, no? So, in typical worked-up and overly sarcastic fashion, I retaliated with my own Facebook update: 'Lisa thinks you lot are a bunch of bastards for going to the pub without her. Can't you wait till she's beaten cancer, you impatient sods?'

*

'Lisa, it's amazing,' said my beautician as she aimed a spray-tanning gun at my tits.

'Told you you'd be impressed,' said Mum. 'And I told *you* there'd be nothing to worry about,' she added, turning to me.

'Really? You reckon?' I asked, still unsure as to whether it was smoke or St Tropez that was being blown up my ass.

'Honestly, darling, I've seen a hundred mastectomies doing this job – and that's one of the best I've sprayed.'

'Well, I'll be sure to tell my surgeon,' I said through pursed lips as I tried not to breathe in the orange fumes.

The thought of my pre-wedding spray-tan had been worrying me for days. Up to this point, the only people who'd seen my cancer-ravaged boob were Smiley Surgeon, Always-Right Breast Nurse, P and those who'd helped me change my dressings, and I wasn't ready to show it off to anyone else. But, having been to the hospital a couple of days previous for Smiley Surgeon to inflate my currently empty tissue-expanding implant, things were finally looking up on the tit front. Because now, I had boobs – *plural*.

I'd been pretty nervous about turning up to see Smiley Surgeon in case he said I was still too swollen to have my implant inflated – aside from anything else, I'd have had an odd-looking, baggy side to the strapless dress I had planned to wear at Jamie's wedding, and visions of my prosthesis shooting out across the dance floor weren't doing much to help. Thankfully, he gave me the go-ahead and pulled out the bike bump (disappointingly, it was more of a huge-needle-and-saline-drip combo) so that I could finally, FINALLY, get rid of the Mastectomy Bra From Hell and my comedy sponge tit (honk honk). It wasn't my old boob, granted, but, in clothes at least, it looked every bit as good. It was round and soft and symmetrical and even a little bit bouncy and, were it not for the fact that I was still singular in the nipple department, it would have been perfect. But even that was due to be rectified a few months down the line in a fascinating process whereby the existing nipple-circle would be twisted into a point, then tattooed to match its non-identical twin. For the meantime, though, I had a fabulous cleavage to enjoy and, after weeks on end of a serious case of the Victor Meldrews, I was damn well going to appreciate it.

Sucking up the worries of how Jamie's wedding guests would react to seeing the cancer-crafted new me (some of whom I hadn't seen since my own wedding – the day on which I looked better than I ever have), I instead set to the remainder of my pre-wedding beauty routine: a long bath, painting my toenails, combing my wig on its stand, face pack, expensive moisturiser . . . What I hadn't bargained for, however, as I ran cotton wool pads over my eyes, was my eyelashes finally giving up the ghost and, with expert comedy timing, dropping out in one blink. I laughed into the cotton wool. Of course they'd fallen out. Waiting until the morning after the wedding just wouldn't have been The Bullshit's way.

Thankfully I was left with four or five stragglers on each lid, onto which we managed to glue emergency false lashes the following morning. Not that lash-gate was the end of my wedding-day cancer-calamities, of course. Minutes before the ceremony, Mum suddenly gestured to my head. 'Christ, Lis, your ears,' she said, panic-stricken. 'Sort your ears out! They're poking out of your wig!'

'Oh for f—,' I held back the expletive, given the occasion. 'I can't pull my wig off *here*,' I said, tutting like a wounded teenager and turning to Dad. 'We're on the front *rowww*; there's all these *peeeople*!'

'Right, come here,' said Dad, leading me off by the elbow to a door to our right and closing it behind us as quietly as the heavy oak would allow.

'Yesss, a mirror,' I squeaked, ripping off my hat and wig in one movement and starting the process of concealing my baldness all over again – this time with my ears tucked away. 'Will that do?'

'Perfect,' said Dad.

'What if it happens during my reading?'

'It won't happen during your reading, you'll be fine.'

'But if it does, right, just point to your ear or something, okay?'

'Okay, stoopid,' he agreed, leading me back out into the ceremony with seconds to spare before Leanne appeared at the top of the aisle, all glittery and gorgeous, like a tiny ballerina inside a musical jewellery box.

In the run-up to the wedding, I was concerned about more than just the physical aspect of how I'd feel – and look – on the big day. P and I had got hitched in the same venue, and I fretted that being there again would upset me, in the same way that looking back at our wedding photos makes us realise how little we knew about our future (and thank God we didn't). But, in fact, none of those things even occurred to me on the day, because the wedding was king; rightfully reigning supreme from Wedding March to first dance. So spectacular was the day that every so often I even forgot I'd got cancer – and that's *damn* high praise.

Missing lashes and wonky wig aside, the important thing was that, for the first time in months, the occasion wasn't about me. Yes, people wanted to ask how I was and tell me they were pleased to see me and lie about how well I looked, but this wasn't my day, so I kept the cancer-talk to a brusque minimum and instead set about the business of being sister of the groom.

And what a groom. Right before my eyes, my kid brother became a man. A confident man; an impressive man; a charming man; a wish-he-was-your-own-brother man. And, thankfully, the kind of man who'd twirl his sister round the dance floor and not take offence when he realised who'd given his best man all those incriminating photocopies.

Seeing Jamie and Leanne get hitched was the prize I'd had my eye on from day one. Every step of The Bullshit up to this point had been geared towards me not just making it there, but having a bloody good time too (mission accomplished). And so, in a way, it felt like the completion of Phase One – now that Jamie and Leanne had become husband and wife, it didn't just mark a new chapter for them, but one for me, too.

Emotional as it was (not least after a few G&Ts), I tried my best not to cry off my false eyelashes – and I did well until Jamie's speech. The speeches are the thing that always get me at any wedding – but this one, of course, was that bit more special. Little git that he is, Jamie really went to town on the emotion, pulling on heart strings like a bell-ringer at St Paul's Cathedral. He said how grateful he was to be marrying into such a lovely family, how stunning the bridesmaids looked, and told how our family had fast become Leanne's fan club – not least Nan and Grandad who, we all knew, would have loved to have been present to witness their union. He told his new wife how he knew from so early on in their relationship that he just *had* to marry her, and promised her mum that he'd always look after her little girl.

And then, to my surprise, he turned to me. 'Sis,' he said, 'thank you for simply being you. The interest you've shown in this wedding when you've had so much more to deal with means the world to us both.' Leanne nodded along, looking at me with beautiful, happy, tear-filled eyes as mine welled up in tandem. 'And we just want you to know,' he continued as he cried, 'that as happy as we feel today, we know that we'll be even happier when you get the all clear.'

Well, that did it. I was ruined. And as soon as I could take my eyes off my extraordinary brother – which, admittedly, was a wee while – I realised that everyone else in the room was ruined, too. There were tissues coming out of every handbag; wet sleeves on every morning suit. But I don't think it was out of sympathy, or sadness at my situation. For me, at least, it was sheer pride in Jamie – wonderful, selfless Jamie who, on the happiest day of his life, had not only refused to allow the shitty, shitty timing of my cancer nightmare to ruin his wedding, but had been so gracious as to acknowledge its presence in such a considerate, compassionate way. Cancer didn't deserve that kind of special treatment. Not even his mid-chemo big sister deserved that kind of special treatment. Nothing that carried even a fraction of negativity had the right to encroach on his and Leanne's wedding, and nobody would have batted a false eyelash if he'd avoided the subject. And yet here we all were, crying off our carefully applied make-up and not giving a stuff.

With our chests puffed out in pride for each other, Jamie and I took our cue to call a halt to the soppy stuff and, mopping up smudged eye-liner and wiping away a plastic eyelash with my tissue, I shook my head in his direction. 'You bastard,' I mouthed, to the retort of a middle-finger salute from my brilliant, brilliant brother.

CHAPTER 19

Something changed

A whole week and no blogging. Well, I think that speaks volumes about how this last chemo cycle has been treating me. Except that it doesn't, really. Not even Shakespeare could explain what it's been like, so instead I'll tell you in a far less eloquent way: it's been fucking horrendous.

My brain has done me the favour of making it impossible to remember just *how* horrific I've felt these past few days, but know this (and know it good): it *was* horrific. And while I might not remember enough to tell you about every pain and symptom and effect, I do remember enough to tell you that I just don't think I can go through it again.

I can hear what you're thinking. I'm almost there . . . nearly done it . . . just one more chemo to go. But that's not just easy for you to say, it's also no comfort whatsoever. It just serves as a reminder that I've got to endure this hell again. 'You're almost there' is indeed a nice thing to say, but it's also the wrong thing to say. I'm aware how much of a bitch that makes me sound, particularly to all the many people who've said that very thing to me lately. (At the expense of whinging even more, this warts-and-all honesty is difficult when you have a compulsive need to

151

feel liked. Last night, unable to sleep, I lay awake drafting letters in my head to all the people I've liked but, I suspect, didn't like me back, asking them what it was about me that made them keep their distance. Does everyone who has a life-threatening illness do this kind of soppy, confessional soul-searching, I wonder?)

But on with the bitchiness. I've had a similar problem with all the messages I've received while I've been laid up this past week. It's a damn good job I was too sick to pick up my phone until last night because, in my state of mind over the last few days, I don't think anyone would have liked the sarcastic replies. ('You've been quiet lately, how's things?' 'How's things? Well, I've still got cancer, I'm in such excruciating pain that I can barely move, I'm suffocating from constant hot flushes, I can't swallow for lumps all over my tongue and, despite being twenty-nine, my mum is having to take me to the loo, which I'm going to pretty often thanks to the fact that I've got the raging shits. So, yeah, things are pretty peachy, thanks.')

I don't like reacting like this, I don't like P and my folks seeing me react like this, and I don't like you reading about me reacting like this. I like to keep as many people as possible sheltered from this stuff, in just the same way that I don't let anyone other than my immediate family see me during my sickest weeks. I'm worried that the sight of me looking like a cross between Voldemort and the Albino Monk will taint people's perception of me in the future, however better I manage to make myself look after The Bullshit is over. My folks have no choice about whether or not they see me that way because, well, they made me. And P signed up for it with the 'support and comfort each other through good times and through troubled times' vow (more fool him). But nobody else should have to be around me when I'm in that state, be it the bitchiness or the sarcasm or the assisted toilet trips or the rotten way I look. So, in weeks like the last one, I tend to hide myself away. And, given my afore-mentioned reaction to innocent 'How are you doing?' messages and 'You're almost there' encouragements, you're probably relieved that I do.

*

Of all the cancer side-effects I'd expected, what I hadn't bargained for was it turning me into a horrible person. But by the time I'd done with Chemo 5, it was more than just the *sight* of myself that I couldn't stand. Ordinarily, I like to think I'm a rather chirpy girl. I smile a lot, I have good manners, I'm nice to people and I avoid confrontation at all costs. But, just as it had ripped the locks from my follicles, chemo seemed to be shredding my good nature, and my mounting frustration with The Bullshit wasn't just being taken out on my pillow – now, other people were getting the brunt of it, too.

Perhaps I'd just run out of cancer pleasantries, and reached the end of my tether when it came to glib conver-sations. Perhaps I'd maxed out on them at the wedding. Whatever it was, I no longer had even the tiniest speck of tolerance for anything that had even the slightest whiff of it'll-be-okay about it. It might be okay in the end, but it wasn't okay now, dammit. I didn't want to be told that there was just one chemo to go. I didn't want to be told how far I'd come, or how well I'd done. All I wanted was to let the world know how shit all of this had been, and how hard done by I was feeling.

On top of all that, it was just starting to dawn on me that a lot of people I knew remained pretty ignorant about what having breast cancer meant for me. I'd had inklings before, after receiving a handful of puzzling, fancy-coming-out-this-weekend texts, but a conversation with Lil finally confirmed it.

'So how was the launch party?' I asked her about some boozy industry do that I'd also received an invitation to. 'See any old faces?'

'Yeah, a few,' she replied. 'It was pretty busy for a school night.'

'Ooh, who?' I asked, after which she reeled off a register-like list of ex-colleagues' names. 'Crikey, I've not seen any of them for ages. So what did you talk about?'

Knowing me as well as she does, Lil knew better than to assume my question meant anything other than 'Did you talk about me?', and she didn't even flinch in giving me my answer.

'Well, that's weird actually,' she began. 'Everyone asked after you, of course, but I couldn't believe how many of them were surprised when I told them you weren't coming to the party.'

'*What?*' I gurned.

'I know, right?'

'But I'm an invalid! A *bald* invalid,' I screeched, tugging at my wig for confirmation and getting agitated beneath my blanket. 'Of course I'm not going to be at the bloody party – I only had chemo last week! Don't they understand?'

With hindsight, I'd later come to realise that of course people didn't understand. Why should they? After all, some folk can lead near-to-normal lives with The Bullshit. But I just wasn't one of them, due to the highly aggressive nature of my Rich-Tea-biscuit-sized tumour that was *this* close to spreading further than my lymph nodes, and the Master Blaster of cancer treatments I was having to kick the shit out of its traces. (I still can't quite believe, by the way, that the biscuit managed to wreak such undetected havoc for so

154

long beneath my left nipple. Because, if my modest tits can disguise that, what the hell else is hidden in my body that I don't know about? Spare change? An old boot? A family of refugees?) But in the heat of that conversation, I was just plain livid. Livid that I'd missed the party and – rather unfairly – livid that not everyone appreciated what that immediate post-chemo week involved.

'They're on another planet,' said Lil, indulging me in my rage by playing along. 'I wanted to say "don't you get it?" but I didn't bother. I mean, where do you start?'

And she was right. Where *do* you start? Because, despite my willingness to write chapter and verse of my cancer story online (which, of course, was hardly compulsory reading for anyone who'd ever come into contact with me), I actually didn't talk about the details with very many people outside of my blog. I guess it was a combination of not wanting them to always equate me with cancer, and wondering whether they really wanted to hear about it in the first place. It's that age-old thing of folk never really being interested in the answer to innocent, throw-away questions like 'how's things?' or 'how was your weekend?'

P, it turned out, was having precisely the same issues with the people around him. Throwing his bag onto the sofa in frustration after work one Monday, he let it be known. 'I'm sick of getting into work on a Monday morning and having to lie about what kind of weekend I've had,' he said. 'I'm losing my patience with it. I always have to say "great, thanks" because nobody wants to hear "oh, I've been nursing my ill wife all weekend", do they?' The majority of P's weekends (and weekdays, for that matter) had, of course, been every bit as shit as mine since The Bullshit chose to trespass on our lovely lives. (With the notable exception of Jamie and Leanne's wedding, obviously. That was worth a hundred weekends.) P wasn't being mean by lying to his colleagues; quite the opposite. Because he, like me, knew better than to tell people the real truth about how our weekend had been. Nobody wants that kind of answer.

As the kind of couple whose diaries used to be packed, it was pretty depressing for us to have had so little fun for so damn long. P and I had always thrived on our dinner meet-ups with mates, pub visits with colleagues and weekends with our family and, as much as we're able to please ourselves without them, doing that with the added weight of The Bullshit does not a memorable few months make. I got pretty tearful about it one Friday night, sparked by my reply of 'April, probably' to an email that asked when I might next be out on the town.

'Where has my normal life gone?' I wailed to P. 'It's like a distant memory. I can't even remember what it's like to feel healthy.'

'I know, darling,' he said, cradling my bald head against his chest. 'We used to have such wonderful weekends.'

'And now you've got to go to work and lie about this one, too.'

'Not necessarily,' said P. 'It is only Friday, after all.'

I craned my neck to look up at his face.

'We could do this weekend *our* way,' he suggested. 'You know, with papers and telly and breakfast in bed. A lovely, quiet, normal weekend.'

'You're on,' I said, shaking his hand to seal the deal. 'We can call round at Tills and Si's too.'

'Absolutely,' P said.

'And then on Sunday let's watch a film and order a curry.'

'Perfect,' he agreed.

'And I'll bake us a cake.'

'Hang on, love,' said P, taken aback by me apparently

volunteering to set foot in the kitchen. 'Let's not get too carried away, eh?'

'Oi,' I shot back, slapping him on the arm. 'I'm going to bake a cake this weekend – and you're going to like it.'

I had been toying with the idea of baking for a few days, keen as I was to find something new to take my mind off the obvious. My nan had baked, and Mum too, but I'd always let the side down with my why-make-what-you-can-buy-in-M&S defence, and the London-specific excuses of being home later than everyone else. But now, with time on my hands and an appetite newly enhanced by steroids, baking seemed as good an option as any.

The newly domesticated me came as something of a surprise to everyone – not least P. The Old Me was happy to tell anyone who'd listen that our kitchen was purely P's territory; New Me was emailing her mates for icing recipes and sending her husband to work with a different Tupperware (*Tupperware!*) of cakes every morning. But I guess a sudden change in the way you spend your time is pretty inevitable in light of a life-altering illness. A friend of Mum's told me that, once her chemo had finished, she took up gardening, having spent her life swerving it – and stunned everyone in the process. But, she said, it just felt natural to her – as baking did to me.

One thing I could never have imagined feeling natural about, however, was the decision that P and I came to later that weekend. At no other time would he have let me get away with it, I'm sure, but with him at work the following Monday, I made a phone call that set in motion a plan to do something so completely out of character that I was certain it would freak out my friends even more than the breast cancer: I was going to get a kitten.

CHAPTER 20

Lonely hearts club

Well, I didn't get a kitten, but I did get a bigger boob. An RSPCA Cat Woman (thankfully no PVC) came round to check out the flat and gave me the go-ahead to pick up my rescue kitten, but the little tyke's gone and got a cold so it looks like the vet's got to hang onto her until she's had her treatment and I've had my final chemo. (And yes, thank you very much, I do see the irony in me having chosen a sick cat.)

Still, after this week's hospital visit for the final part of my implant inflation, it might not be altogether a bad thing that I didn't have a kitten crawling all over me and my painful left boob. And if you believe that, you've not been reading my blog long enough. In truth, the kitten – just like the baking and the blogging – has been a cheerful distraction from just how panicked, worried and want-to-run-away scared I am about the next chemo. And now she's not able to come home yet, I'm back to fretting and crying uncontrollably. So that 'might not be altogether a bad thing' line is, of course, a load of toot. I'd much rather be crying about a kitten having jumped on my sore tit than the prospect of another horrific chemo, and facing up to the reality of the damage it's done to me so far, physically and emotionally.

But back to business. The falsie is actually more tender than painful now, and no bloody wonder considering what it's been put through. To compensate for the implant-shrinking effects of radiotherapy, Smiley Surgeon inflated it to a size slightly larger than my right one. Not to the point where anyone other than me, P and Smiley Surgeon (the only other man allowed to mess with my boobs) would notice, mind, but it still feels like I've got a bowling ball stuffed down the left side of my T-shirt.

This implant, however, won't be sticking around for much longer and, to be honest, I'm glad. As brilliant as it is to have a lovely round boob and a killer cleavage again, it's not at all comfortable. I can feel the plastic edge of the implant underneath my skin, and the valve attached to it that Smiley Surgeon uses for inflation doesn't just dig in, but can be easily located by an ugly-looking bruise. But thankfully all of that will be a thing of the past in April when I have my next lot of surgery. At the same time as creating a new nipple, Smiley Surgeon will also replace my plastic boob with the Gold Standard of falsies: a silicone implant.

I was hoping it could all be done a bit sooner than April, but apparently I'm underestimating the effects of radiotherapy and how long it'll take for me to recover from it. Smiley Surgeon has clearly been trying to make me realise this for the last three or four appointments I've had with him but, frankly, I've just not had the space in my head to deal with it. But with my final chemo tomorrow and radiotherapy not far off, I finally took in all the things he was saying about how tired, queasy and sore it was going to make me feel, and how it was going to take a fair few weeks of getting over before I'd be surgery-ready again.

I adore Smiley Surgeon. I'm so eager to please that I save my best brave face for my appointments with him, I look up to him as though he were a rock star and I hang on every last word he says. I love him. Not like *that*. It's not a crush. I'm much more goofy than flirty when I'm around him – actually, I'm an embarrassing suck-up. And anyway, the love's not just reserved for Smiley Surgeon, but also for his sidekick, Always-Right Breast Nurse. Batman and Robin have got nothing on these two – holy smoke, they're incredible. So often, medical professionals know all the facts of a condition, but lack the emotional under-standing of how to deal with their patients. Not these two. They're the perfect mix of matter-of-fact and caring, and they always – *always* – hit the right note.

Something P and I particularly love about them is the fact that they'd got the pair of us sussed from the very beginning. We come as a team, P and I, and Smiley Surgeon and Always-Right Breast Nurse were quick to recognise it. They always ask how *we* are. The *you* in 'how did you find the last chemo?' is collective. When there's a decision to make, they ask what both of us think about it. And how can you not fall in love with people like that?

But there's a bigger reason for my adulation. These people saved my life! Every time Smiley Surgeon shakes my hand, I want to grab him and hug him instead. With every bit of advice he gives me, I want to reply with an eloquent response that lets him know just how brilliant I think he is. I want to make him dinner and bake him cakes and write him poems and nominate him for awards and commission a statue of him and shout from the rooftops of London about what a bloody marvellous genius of a man he is. But even I know that none of that's appropriate (well, apart from the cake-baking, perhaps). So until I find a better way to express my gratitude, I'm going to keep acting goofy and sucking up and grinning like an idiot at every appointment. Maybe he'll even start calling me Smiley Patient. I only hope I'll come to love my kitten as much as I love my surgeon.

*

'This one's purring like a good'un,' said Busby, swapping the comatose ball of fluff I was holding with the decidedly lively tortoiseshell kitten she'd picked up.

'Oh, okay, I see. So that's purring, is it?' I queried, puzzled by the vibrating feline.

'Good Lord, woman, you really don't know a thing about cats, do you?'

'Well, I'm about to find out,' I said. 'Cos I'm having this one.'

'Good choice, bird, good choice,' confirmed Busby.

'Eh up, toffee-paws,' I said to the tiny cat, turning and lifting her so that we were looking eye-to-eye. 'You okay to come home with me, then? I've no idea what I'm doing, like, but we'll figure it out.'

The kitten stared back blankly, still purring like a good'un.

'I'll take that as a yes.'

'I still can't believe you're really doing this,' said Busby, eyeing up the other cats yet to be rescued. 'You're not the Mac we all knew!'

'You've got that right,' I confirmed. 'I just never imagined it would involve becoming a pet owner. I'm as surprised as you are.'

I'd better give you some background here. Among my friends, I've always been known as 'Anti-Animal Mac'. If someone ever showed me a picture of their cat/dog/bunny/whatever, I was physically unable to produce an 'aah', instead making some nice-pet-but-I'd-rather-see-it-between-a-burger-bun crack and reiterating to anyone who'd listen that I. Was. Not. An. Animal. Person. Me getting a pet was about as likely as me getting breast cancer. So why the sudden decision to do it?

Frankly, I blame Tills. Which, unfairly, is often my answer

to those kinds of questions. ('You're drunk at two o'clock on a weekday?' 'You spent *how* much on a handbag?' Etc.) But this time, it kind of is. Because, on going round to theirs one weekend for a dinner party with our mates Polly and Martin, we were greeted by the teeny-tiny RSPCA rescue kitten that she and Si had just given a home to. And the damn thing won me over. It was the first animal ever to show a favourable interest in me (and vice versa), and it got me thinking how great it would be to have some company while I was spending so much time in the flat on my own. (And beyond, of course – a cat's not just for Christmas. Or cancer.)

'You should totally get one,' said Tills, as her miniature, picture-perfect kitten curled up in the palm of my hand. 'Look how much Clarry likes you.' She nudged P, encouraging him to agree.

'I've got to say, I never thought I'd see the day that you held a cat,' he said. 'If only your nan could see you now.' (Nan was famous for the anti-cat devices in her garden. Barbed wire round the top of the fence, Olbas oil on the path, water-filled milk bottles ready to soak trespassers at a nanosecond's notice. Even when clearing out the garden after she'd died, Dad narrowly missed impaling himself on a wooden stump that Nan had hammered nails into the side of – a bad-ass weapon she'd doubtless knocked together in Grandad's shed while a home-made crumble cooked in the oven.)

I fluttered my eyelashes in P's direction. 'What do you reckon?'

'Yes! Do it! Do it! Do it!' squealed Tills. 'Our cats can be mates!'

'You're not really serious, are you?' asked Si.

'I dunno. I think I am.'

'Ha! Polly! Get in here! Mac's getting a cat!' Tills shrieked.

'What?' said Polly, appearing in a stunned flash from the kitchen. 'Why?'

'Well, y'know, I guess I'm just getting a bit lonely in the flat all day on my own,' I reasoned, apologetically. 'It's company, innit.'

'Well, good on you,' she agreed. 'They're *amazing* company. Calming, too.'

'It's *perfect* timing,' added Tills, still ridiculously over-excited. 'Because by the time it's ready to head outside, you will be too.'

'Ooh and I can fit you a cat-flap,' said Si, ever keen to tackle some DIY.

'Shit, are we really doing this?' asked P. 'I mean, I'm cool with it – I just can't believe you are.'

'Me neither,' I mumbled, shaking my head. 'What the hell's got into me?'

'Sod all that,' said Martin. 'What are you going to call it?'

'Ooh, now there's a question,' I pondered.

Later that night, after an evening of my animated mates listing all the pros and cons of getting a kitten, I actually found myself feeling a bit sad that there wasn't one waiting for me when we got home. Getting into bed, P made the fatal error of saying he 'wouldn't say no' if I decided to adopt a cat of my own. And so it was kind of his fault, too. But mostly, of course, it was The Bullshit's doing: all the endless being-ill-at-home lark had become so lonely and boring that even I, Chief Animal Hater, was getting a pet.

My family were as baffled by my decision as my friends. After all, the last they knew of me caring for an animal was Miss Ellie, the goldfish I used to stir around in its bowl with a wooden spoon when I was two. But despite their surprise, they were all on board for one reason: already, even before bringing her home, the kitten had made me happy. Planning her arrival was something I cheerfully sank my teeth into – within days, I had the bowls and beds and litter tray and scratching post all in position (and all complementary to the décor – sheesh, I hadn't changed *that* much), and the weekly Sainsbury's order had been amended to include all the things a soon-to-be-spoiled kitten might need. It was my new baking substitute – a brand-new tactic to take my mind off The Bullshit in a week when I'd otherwise have been climbing-up-the-walls terrified about my final chemo.

'Are you sure you're okay with this?' I asked P while cheerfully unpacking enough Whiskas to feed all the cats in south-west London.

'Whatever makes you smile this much can't be a bad thing,' he said.

The next few pre-chemo days were spent explaining my kitten-decision to other friends. To them, me becoming a pet owner was such an about-turn that I feared they'd be expecting a totally different girl to walk into the pub the following spring. I could see it now – them asking me pop-quiz questions to confirm my identity and checking my handbag to see whether I still carried around a pen to correct any punctuation, spelling or grammar errors I came across. And so, ensuring my cap was doffed to the Old Me, I predictably chose a Beatles-referencing name for my kitten to make them realise that, pet aside, I was still me. Besides, Sgt Pepper is a far better name than Apostrophe.

CHAPTER 21

One step beyond

November 2008

I do like an excuse for a celebration, and here's a corker for you: I HAVE FINISHED CHEMO. Feel free to break into applause.

Actually, the celebrations only lasted as long as Friday evening, when P and I counted down the last millilitres of drugs running through my drip, said our emotional goodbyes to the nurses (after plying them with home-made fairy cakes) and bid a final, fond fuck-off to the chemo room. When we got back to the car, we allowed ourselves five minutes of exhausted tears (as opposed to worried tears or downhearted tears or frightened tears — just as Eskimos have their numerous types of snow, cancer patients have their numerous types of crying) before taking a detour on the way home to pick up Sgt Pepper, adding a nice full stop to the end of our chemo nightmare. (Told you I should have named her after a punctuation mark.)

But as celebrations go, that was about it. And I can't help feeling that it's all a bit lacking. Granted, I've hardly been up to raising my arms in joy since Friday; I have, inevitably, been a bit on the rubbish side (to put it exceptionally mildly) and doing congas round the flat isn't all that simple when you're out-on-your-arse ill and feeling like you've been victim to a gangland kneecapping. I look like it, too. You bruise like a peach when you're on chemo and, thanks to the addition of an eager-to-clamber-up-for-a-cuddle kitten, the bruises and scratches make it look like I've spent the past week self-harming.

Me, Tills, Busby, Weeza and the boys let off a few fireworks in the back garden the night before Chemo 6, which I think was a fitting ceremony. Or at least it was until a normally-volume-challenged neighbour (who thought it acceptable to sit in her garden all summer long holding court about her post-breastfeeding chafing nipples) cut the festivities short by pulling out the sleeping-baby excuse. I wish I'd have been quick enough to retaliate because I'm pretty certain that, in Excuses Top Trumps, cancer beats baby.

*

It was impossible to know how best to mark the end of chemo. Plant a tree? Unveil a plaque? Throw a party? Run naked down Oxford Street? There's always the Louboutins, mind you, but right now I fear they'd buckle under the bulk of my bloated frame. But with radiotherapy just around the corner, I questioned whether or not it was even appropriate to mark the end of a shitty few months when there were numerous other struggles to contend with. And so, short of setting fire to the fence with a Catherine wheel and renting a motorhome for next year's Glastonbury (or Middle-class-tonbury, as we soon renamed it), P and I bowed out of any commemorations and concentrated our efforts on the newest member of our family instead.

With hindsight, picking up Sgt Pepper on the way home from chemo might not have been the smartest idea we've ever had. Add a terrified kitten to a woozy cancer patient and a husband who doesn't know which of the two to look after, and you've got yourself a recipe for a rather bizarre evening. As soon as we got her home, we limited Sgt Pepper to the kitchen, figuring that it was best for her to get used to her new home room by room rather than all at once. And so we set ourselves the same boundaries for a few hours, sitting on the kitchen floor and watching baffled as a black-and-gold fuzzball ricocheted from one skirting board to another.

'Is Lisa all right?' Mum asked P in a phone call that night.

'She's on the kitchen floor.'

'Oh my God, has she collapsed? Do you need us there?'

'Oh nonono, she's on the floor with the cat. It's a bloody nightmare.'

'Um, didn't she ought to be in bed instead of the kitchen floor?' enquired Mum.

'Honestly, she's okay at the moment. She can't walk around much. But she wants to make sure Sgt Pepper settles in okay.'

'And has she?'

'Well, she pissed up the skirting board as soon we got her here and she's been going pretty mental since.'

'Riiight.'

'We don't know what we're doing, Jane. I think we've made a terrible mistake.'

P and I wondered whether you could equate adopting a kitten with bringing home a new-born baby from hospital – the excitement of having her quickly turned to flat panic when we realised that neither of us knew what the hell to do with our new arrival. And, with the knowledge that Chemo 6's 'buggery bit' would hit within the next twenty-four hours, we were desperate to make Sgt Pepper feel comfortable before I felt the opposite. In the end, we went against the keep-her-to-one room advice, and were pleased we did. Because the moment she caught sight of the living room, and the linen-lined basket we'd prepared for her, she immediately mellowed, melting into her pink blanket like a marshmallow in a chocolate fondue, after which I took my cue to do the same in my own bed.

And that, in a nutshell, was as much of a hooray as I enjoyed once the final dribble of chemo had dripped its way into my veins. I had half expected there to be an emancipatory Nicole Kidman moment when I walked out of the hospital that day; throwing my arms out wide and raising myself up on my tiptoes in release from the shackles of my ordeal (though I reckon even chemo has the torture-edge on being married to Tom Cruise). But, with a meagre few hours of smugness before my body was turned to bilge and my mind was turned to mud for the final time, P and I were reluctant to revel for long.

In all truth, though, there were more reasons than the chemo-ills for my lack of enthusiasm in terms of moving on. Because, in my final consultation with Glamorous Assistant before my treatment began that day, I shamed myself by asking her for a referral to a therapist – yet another thing that had featured on my list of Things I Said I'd Never Do.

'I don't like asking this,' I told her, 'but I think it's necessary . . .'

'Go on,' she said, clasping her hands together and swivelling her chair a little more in my direction.

'Well, a while back you mentioned that there was a therapist at the hospital, and I think—'

'Not a problem,' she interrupted, saving me the indignity of having to admit to anything other than complete mental strength. 'I'll refer you today, and I'm sure you'll hear from them next week.'

'Thank you,' I said. 'It's not that I'm depressed or anything, right? I just think I need some help to make sense of all of this.'

'It's perfectly normal, Lisa,' she assured me. 'Many patients do the same – there's an awful lot to take in.'

'You're not kidding,' I replied.

'Honestly, don't worry. You'll be pleased you did it,' she said.

And so, in typical, prematurely panicking fashion, I immediately brushed aside any hope of end-of-chemo celebrations and set to fretting about therapy instead, even before I'd made an appointment.

'Why can't I just enjoy the moment?' I said to P in bed that night. 'I thought we'd be cracking open the champagne tonight, but instead I'm worrying about what's next.'

'That's pretty much your nature though, isn't it, babe?' he said, correctly.

'But it's like I'm a masochist or something. It's like I'm dead-set on pissing on my own bonfire.'

'Can you stop being so hard on yourself please?' P pleaded. 'I mean, let's be honest – there's a shit few days coming up, but after that things are going to get better.'

'Hmpf,' I exhaled.

'Come off it. They *are*. And going to therapy is a step in the right direction. It's a good thing. It's all part of the cure.'

'You're always the sodding voice of reason, aren't you?' I whinged, approaching my descent into the bitch-mode that came with feeling so depressingly unwell.

'I am, yeah,' he said. 'So you'd better bloody listen to me.'

The subsequent few days were predictably hellish. The accumulative build-up of the drugs in my body had restricted my movement so much that I was confined to my bedroom, feeling like more of a cancer patient than ever with P and my folks again peering down at me with pity in their eyes, and Mum having to help me to the toilet every time I needed to go. With little voice to shout with and zero energy to make my own way out of bed, I'd knock on the wall above the headboard or the door beside the bed whenever I needed something, and someone would come skipping in.

'We should have got you a bell to ring,' Mum said.

'You'd have been sick of the sound of it,' I whimpered.

Dad adopted his usual position, curled up beside me for our now-routine private father-daughter chats and as much of a cuddle as I could manage, and we'd natter into the night about family and football and whatever we could think of that was a world away from The Bullshit. 'Can we still do this even when you're not ill, doofus?' he asked.

'Damn right. I'll be sitting on your knee even when I'm fifty,' I promised him.

Physically, Chemo 6 was undoubtedly worse than Chemo 5 had been. The accrued level of toxic liquids pumping their way around my useless limbs made even the simplest movement – turning over in bed, lifting a cup of tea – feel like a punishing endurance test. But this round, at least, the realisation that I wouldn't be having to endure it all over again in three weeks' time made it infinitely easier to deal with mentally. So even though it felt like my legs were breaking and I was looking progressively more like Fester Addams, in a funny way, it didn't matter half as much. Because, as I said to Mum, Dad and Jamie in a triumphant text message on my way home from the hospital: CHEMO IS OVER.

CHAPTER 22

I got my head checked

Well, I've done it. I've crossed the line. Turned to the dark side. I am now a woman in therapy. Actually, they don't call it 'therapy' at my hospital. It's 'counselling'. But since I'm not fond of either of those words, I'm going to call it Brain Training instead. A bit like on the Nintendo DS, but in this version they don't make you do maths, count syllables or draw kangaroos.

Clearly, I went into this with very little knowledge of therapy. The little I do know I've learned from Tony Soprano, and I'm not convinced he's the best example of how to act. Even after this week's session, I'm still not sure how much I know about therapy. But now, at least, I don't think it really matters. Because what is there to know, other than whether or not you like it, and whether or not you think it can do you any good? As it goes, I'm sold already. Although I must admit that while I was sitting in the waiting room, any excuse to do a runner would have done: I was having a bad wig day; I didn't have any tissues; my chipped nails would give the wrong impression. In the end I took my mind off it by reading the posters in the waiting room and, just as I spotted one calling for patients to judge a poetry competition and not-so-surreptitiously balanced on my chair to take a photo of the contact details (i.e., just as I reached new lows of spoddy and uncool), in walked my therapist. Let's call him Mr Marbles, since it's his job to find them.

Mr Marbles steadfastly ignored my pleasantries about what kind of week he'd had as we walked along the oddly familiar corridor to his office. This déjà vu suddenly made sense when I heard the instantly recognisable sound of Crap FM coming from the cupboard-like room several doors down. A sneaky look as I walked by left me surprised to discover that the figure in there, surrounded by boxes of grey syrups and tapping her feet to Destiny's Child, was not, in fact, Wig Man, but an equally bored-looking and lacking-in-job-satisfaction Wig Woman. I giggled on my way into the Brain Training room, then stopped when I realised it might make me look too jovial and unworthy of free NHS therapy.

The next thing I knew it was fifty minutes later, I had a handful of crumpled tissues, redder eyes than I went in with and was listening to Mr Marbles read out the notes he'd written throughout the seemingly lightning-speed session. By heck, you don't half get going when someone gives you the opportunity to talk about yourself. Poor sod could hardly get a peep in. When I did finally give him the chance to speak, though, every single thing he said further convinced me that the Brain Training is a good idea.

Just like everyone else I've encountered at the hospital, Mr Marbles is brilliant. Again, I felt that now-familiar, wonderful, über-professional mix of total understanding and a means-business determination to help. He's sensible and serious, but not to the point of being unable to crack a smile. He puts you at immediate ease, doesn't pass judgement and never lets his face give away what he's thinking. Plus he wears corduroy slacks. Of course he wears corduroy slacks. I'd have been disappointed if he didn't wear corduroy slacks.

During the session, we spoke about survival instincts and concerns and expectations and outlooks and fears. I talked endlessly, sobbed and apologised a fair bit. He nodded, scribbled notes in an orange file and revealed that the best-known way to feel instantly better is to make sure your husband buys you a pair of Louboutins. (He also identified humour as one of my coping strategies. I suspect it's more sarcasm.) The whole coping-strategy shizzle is a funny one, though. Not least because the words 'coping strategy' sound like something David Brent would say. But, semantics aside, I reckon that, in a roundabout way, I'd already realised that I had a few coping strategies up my sleeve. I'd just been calling them 'projects', is all. (Yep, we're back to the old blogging/baking/kitten equation.)

Naturally, that conversation backed me into a better-tell-him-about-the-blog corner. And so I did. I told him how often I posted, the kind of things I blog about, what writing it has meant to me, how it's helped my family and friends understand my experience of breast cancer and how it's made me realise that I want to keep writing, even when The Bullshit is a distant memory. (I didn't call it The Bullshit, by the way. Probably best to save the expletives until session three or four.) Mr Marbles asked how people had responded to the blog, whether I'd ever reread it from the beginning (I haven't) and how I think it'd make me feel if I were reading, as opposed to writing, it. I started to worry that he'd ask for the web address, too, but (a) I'm sure that'd be against some sort of Counsellor's Code and (b) after spending all day listening to people's neuroses, the last thing he'll want to do when he gets home is read 60,000 words of the same. The man's got telly to watch and wine to drink and slacks to iron.

*

As I'd moaned to P before my therapy appointment, my frustration was growing over my inability to stop peering round corners, trying to guess when the next shit-pie would come hurtling towards me. I simply couldn't – or wouldn't allow myself to – pause for a moment to bask in the glorious achievement of having seen off an almost impossibly traumatic, exhausting, immune-system-destroying, tumour-killing, total git of a course of chemo. Because, God knows, that was my time to lap it up. Instead, I brushed all of that aside in favour of fretting about another issue altogether, and forcing my husband to stay up until 2.30 a.m. the night before therapy so we could talk it out.

One of the main reasons (*the* main reason?) I asked for a therapy referral was that I was worrying about the process of moving into a life of non-treatment and eventual remission; specifically, a life that was very different from the one I left behind when I heard the words 'signs consistent with breast cancer'. A significant concern stemmed from the fact that, pre-Bullshit, everything for P and I was geared towards having a baby. But suddenly, thanks to the cancer-creating effects of oestrogen on my body, everything was geared towards us *not* having a baby. As I've mentioned before, it wasn't as though P and I had never before been forced to consider a childless life; it's something we've given more thought to than most. But now, knowing that the no-kids issue would no longer be an 'if', it created another hurdle for us to negotiate, and I spent more time than I care to admit worrying about what to do next.

I know it was rather a daft thing to be fretting about given the circumstances, but I bemoaned the deviation from my carefully scripted Grand Life Plan. And, in turn, I was frustrated with myself for allowing such a ridiculous thing to bother me so much when, surely, the bigger worry at hand should have been the fertility issue itself? My tendency to plan had gone too far. I mean, hell, not even getting breast cancer could teach me that it was impossible to map out my life – which was why I needed a therapist to kick me up the arse instead.

As I explained to Mr Marbles, I wasn't worried about whether or not I'd be content and fulfilled in the future – once the health stuff fell into place, I knew I'd have all the right ingredients for a very happy life. It was more a case of worrying that, if P and I weren't going to have kids (and with adoption agencies hardly gasping to add a cancer patient to their books), then what, exactly, *were* we going to do? What was in the Grand Life Plan now? And I wasn't alone in thinking like this. In our 2.30 a.m. talk-athon, P revealed that he had been having much the same thoughts (match made in heaven or what?).

'It's not just about us though, is it?' I said to P.

'How do you mean?' he replied, puzzled.

'Well, your mum and dad,' I continued. '*My* mum and dad! Maybe it's more of a shame for them than it is for us? They must have expected grandchildren, right?'

'God, yeah, of course. And our mates will have expected it from us, too. They're all at it, after all.'

We were in that happy stage of our lives where the people around us were endlessly announcing engagements, weddings, pregnancies and christenings, and P and I are very good at the business of being genuinely interested, enthusiastic and delighted on their behalves. (Yeah, we're lovely like that. We should hire ourselves out. Rent-a-Reaction.)

But now there were no kids on the table, we didn't want people to be anxiously anticipating how we'd react to their news, or for them to feel they had to water down their joy

175

because of us. Yes, with every pregnancy that was announced there might be a wistful window into what could have been. Yes, it might hurt and we might shed a few tears over it behind closed doors. But we're not the kind of people who'd ruin anyone's fun with the unfortunate reality of our situation. So, to prepare ourselves and be ready at a moment's notice to dish out all the right handshakes, back-slaps, hugs and congratulations, we set to making a mental list of all the friends and family we were expecting to announce baby news over the next few years, and in what order. It may have been crazy, but it made us feel better in that moment. Because, when you've had as huge a shock in your lives as P and I had, it's an instinctive reaction to anticipate where the next one's coming from.

I wish I could tell you that our worrying stopped there, at the impending few years. But I'm assuming you know me better than that by now, so I might as well admit to the following conversation.

'It's the dinner parties I worry about,' said P, now breaking into our stash of emergency Maltesers. 'When all of our mates have kids and we don't, will we have nothing to add to the conversation?'

'You're right, yeah,' I agreed. 'Like childcare and tuition fees and the latest toys.'

'I just don't want to stop being part of their lives because of this, you know? Because some people are defined by their children – like your parents and my parents. So I don't want us to be defined by *not* having had them.'

'And I don't want anyone to patronise us because of it, either. I don't want people to tilt their heads and say, "Ah. P and Lisa. Lovely couple. Couldn't have kids. Shame." Like that awful dinner party in *Bridget Jones's Diary* or something.'

'You know what pisses me off?' continued P, his cheeks puffed out with honeycomb balls. 'How some people used to say to me, "Oh you wouldn't understand until you were married" – that kind of stuff. What? So I wouldn't understand what it's like to love someone so much that they're your whole world, and you'd be completely devastated by their loss? It's fucking ridiculous.'

'But nobody would say that to us about kids, surely?'

'Hmpf, I wouldn't be so sure. I've heard that sentence a couple of times before,' continued P, increasingly agitated. 'And I never – *never* – want to hear it again.'

To put it simply, we just didn't want people feeling sorry for us. Because there was nothing to feel sorry for and because, despite everything, I don't know many people with as happy a relationship as me and P. And, kids or no kids, that's quite the lucky break.

I was quick to communicate all of that to Mr Marbles.

'And you're married, yes?' he asked.

'I am; to P,' I answered.

'And are you able to talk to him about any fears or difficulties?'

'Yes. Absolutely. Yes, of course. He's wonderful,' I said, a little too enthusiastically.

'Well, that's good,' he concluded.

'It *is* good,' I continued. 'It's better than good. It's perfect. I want you to know how lucky I feel to be in that kind of marriage.'

Just as I didn't want therapy to force me to deconstruct my relationships with my folks or my family or my friends, I refused to do it with my relationship with P, either. I wasn't there for that kind of stuff – and I wanted to make it clear from the off.

'The thing is,' I said to Marbles, 'I haven't come here

because I don't have anyone else to talk to. I've got plenty of people to talk to. Honestly, aside from this cancer stuff I really am exceptionally lucky. I just don't want those people to have to hear all of this.'

'And why is that?' he asked, scribbling in the notebook that was leaning on his crossed legs.

'They've heard enough of my whinging.'

'It's not whinging,' he said abruptly.

'Well, whatever it is, I don't want them to hear it. There are things I need to discuss here that I never want them to be party to. They've had enough heartbreak from me, and they don't deserve any more. Plus, I couldn't handle the guilt of offloading onto them.'

We continued to talk about the guilt I was feeling generally – about getting cancer in the first place, about the time everyone had given up to look after me, about the hopelessly defeatist things I used to say in the darkest throes of sickness – and about the disappointingly empty anticlimax of finishing chemotherapy.

'Did you do anything to mark the end of chemo?' asked Marbles.

'Well we got the kitten.' I shrugged. 'But more than that, no. I didn't feel it appropriate to celebrate.'

'How so?'

'Well, it would have been a bit like throwing a party once you've been released from months of being held captive: you're ecstatic to be out, but nonetheless completely traumatised by what you've been through.'

'That's a good analogy,' he said, and I beamed at his compliment in the same arse-licky way I would with Smiley Surgeon.

'Besides,' I continued, 'it's not over yet, is it?'

Whether or not it was really the conclusion, the goal I had

178

been aiming for was not the end of chemo, but instead the last bit of reconstructive surgery the following April – the time, I assumed, at which I'd finally begin to feel like my healthy old self again. Plus, my breast cancer road began with the removal of my left boob, and my finish-line medal was the chance to get it back for good. Of course, the reality is that reconstructive surgery isn't actually the end. In fact, where grade-three breast cancer is concerned, there is no 'end' to speak of. And it was really frustrating to realise that there was never going to be a clearly defined finale to punctuate that period of my life. Especially as you know how much I like to punctuate.

If you don't count the surgery, it all starts and ends so differently (and by 'ends' I mean 'fizzles out'). Life-changing and heartbreaking and terrifying and shocking and dark and disastrous as the moment is, there's a ceremony around being told that you have breast cancer. There's a sombre appointment in a specialist's office with all manner of people on hand to answer your questions, hand you a tissue and bring you a cup of tea. You get sent cards, flowers, chocolates, books, toiletries, DVDs, magazines, poems, soft toys (if cancer has an upside, surely this is it). You have a seemingly endless stream of visitors. You become the topic of conversation in the offices and pubs and kitchens and inboxes and Facebook walls that you're suddenly absent from. And it's the weirdest thing. Nothing is more disconcerting. But there's no doubting that it all marks a definite, no-question, breast-cancer-begins-here starting point.

So, by that token, wouldn't it be only fair to have a breast-cancer-ends-here moment? A moment when you can make happier calls and send I'm-free emails and get more flowers and receive celebratory 'you beat The Bullshit' cards? But I think we've already established that nothing about cancer is fair. Cancer is an attention-seeking, party-pooping bitch. It takes over. It takes your hair, your confidence, your social life, your immune system, your figure (the least it could do is make you thin, for fuck's sake), your energy, your taste buds, your sense of smell, your sex life. And just when you think it's done as much as it possibly can, it takes away your chance to celebrate the end of it all.

Once you've had cancer, no medical professional will ever say the words 'cancer free' to you. You're too much of a risk, and they'd be opening themselves up to a world of trouble if it turned out that the cancer was sneakily plotting a return, as it often does. That's why the word 'remission' comes in so handy. And so, pitifully few cancer experiences end neatly with a concern-free CT scan or a clear set of test results or a finish-it-off bit of surgery, as I pretended mine would. There's a lifetime of tablets, appointments, tests, scans, mammograms. And while it's hugely comforting that the NHS doesn't just spit you back out as soon as you've had the necessary treatment, it does seem like a case of once a cancer patient, always a cancer patient.

I like a clear finish, not a fade-out (it's the reason I've always preferred 'Please Please Me' to 'Love Me Do'). I appreciate a wrap-up; a good, old-fashioned full stop. Loose ends don't sit well with me. But this fade-out was, I had to concede, another thing that I simply had no control over. I couldn't create a false conclusion to The Bullshit just to satisfy my need for closure. Some things, I guess, aren't meant to reach a proper finale (hell, there's never a final episode of *Coronation Street* and that's never bothered me). I was still determined to punctuate the passing of those strange few months, mind. It just looked like that chapter would have to finish with . . . instead of.

CHAPTER 23

To boldly go

Something weird happened yesterday. Either I had my radio-therapy planning appointment or I was abducted by aliens. For an actually-pretty-serious hospital appointment, I found this one the most entertaining yet. It was like a cross between *Star Trek* and the 'Cartman Gets an Anal Probe' episode of *South Park*. Except instead of a satellite up my jacksie, I've been given three very questionable-looking tattoos on my chest. I'd tell you that they're preferable to an anal probe but actually I'm not so sure, given that I now look like someone's been playing dot-to-dot in my cleavage with a blue biro.

The rest of the planning appointment was much more space age, thankfully. You gown up and lie topless on a black leather bed (not as S&M as it sounds, I assure you) in the middle of a huge, futuristic room that could easily have dual use as a record-ing studio on the *Starship Enterprise*. Then the radiographer versions of Captain Kirk and Uhura come out from behind the mixing desk to press buttons on a bunch of different computers that whirr around your body before fixing you into an unnatural position (again, not in a kinky way) that you've got to stay in for the next fifty minutes, and for each subsequent twenty-minute radiotherapy session. And who'd have thought that years of cheesy discos could prepare you for such an event? Because, for the next six weeks, you'll be able to find me on a hospital bed doing a stationary version of the 'YMCA'. Actually it's more like the YM. Y with the left arm, M with the right. (And it's a good job, really – I've always found C and A to be the trickier parts of the dance.)

So there you lie, unable to laugh out loud at the ridiculousness of the situation because the *Enterprise* crew has warned you not to move. And considering the intricate, no-margin-for-error measuring they're having to do to make sure the rays will always target the right area, I guess it's fair enough. It was all rulers, angles and trigonometry, with all kinds of crew members looking serious, shouting out numbers and talking to each other in a complicated, technical language (Klingon, perhaps?).

Now don't get me wrong, they're very lovely, but the radio-therapy staff are completely different to the chemo crowd. The 'therapy' part of each treatment fools you into thinking that the two must somehow be linked, when actually they're at opposite ends of the cancer stratosphere. In chemo, you can have a bit of a giggle with the nurses while they're hooking you up to your drip. But radiotherapy seems to be that bit more serious – more of an exact science – so joking about with the staff (while you're lying on the bed, at least) is a bit like knocking the back of Steve Davis's snooker cue when he's about to pot the black for the World Championship.

Anyway, after the acid-trip of hospital appointments, we're finally all systems go for radiotherapy to begin a week on Monday. And, this Friday aside, I don't have to go back to the hospital until then. Result or what? I fear I'll get withdrawal symptoms and start showing up there out of habit. And get this – later this week, I'm even getting the chance to dust off my glad rags to go to an awards do with work. I know! An actual night out! (Is it just me, or are things beginning to look up?) Thankfully there's still one dress in my wardrobe I can fit into. Quite a busty little number, as it goes. I'm secretly hoping someone will pull me to one side and say, 'Excuse me, love, but you've got a biro mark in your cleavage.'

*

With chemo out of the way, and my health steadily improving before radiotherapy kick-off, there opened a small window in which I could enjoy my mini-break from The Bullshit. And, after five months of enforced sobriety and cancer-captivity, a couple of long-scheduled nights out proved beautiful timing. The first was a yearly industry awards ceremony at which my company had arranged two tables. Anticipating what a big deal this otherwise-standard night would be for me, my boss Kath kept me posted for at least a week with daily emails on what everyone else from the office would be wearing, and arranged a car to collect me on the night.

'How are you feeling about this, then?' she asked on the way over.

I bit my lip and furrowed my brow. 'Nervous. Really nervous.'

'Nothing to be nervous about,' quipped Kath. 'You know how lovely everyone is, and they're all really looking forward to seeing you.'

'I know,' I said. 'But the wig. I know a lot of them saw it that day when I came into the office, but you know what it's like at these things – everyone looking across tables to seek out their ex-colleagues and gawp at who's wearing what and who's put on weight and all that. I just hope I don't see anyone I know, is all.'

'Well, I've put you next to Keith,' she assured me. 'And he's on strict instructions to take you under his wing and look after you.'

'Ah! Nice one!' I exclaimed, perking up – Keith being the office Good Guy, and the perfect colleague to be sat next to at these occasions.

'Mind you, by "looking after you" he'll probably take that as his cue to get you roaring drunk.'

'Ha, well it won't take much,' I said. 'Better keep an eye on me, eh?'

Inside the venue, I walked tentatively over to the corner commandeered by our company, tottering precariously on patent heels as though I were four and trying on my mum's stilettos for the first time. Keith immediately bounded over. 'Lynchy!' he roared, his arms wide open as if The Fonz had just walked into the room. 'You look ace. Come here!' And he grabbed me for a hug so tight I feared my wig would get irretrievably caught in his watch strap. 'Ayy, Sarah, look who it is!' he said, turning to our equally chirpy colleague and pulling her in for a group hug. 'It's Lynchy! She's back in the fold!'

I appreciated Keith's enthusiasm, and how it seemed to be spreading to everyone else in our corner. People rubbed my shoulders and slapped me on the back and fibbed about how well I looked, and – in light of having read about Sgt Pepper on my blog – a colleague handed me a gift of a cat-shaped doorstop. I should have known that this lovely lot would make me feel instantly comfortable. Nobody talked about cancer, nobody looked at me funny, nobody avoided me . . . it was just a normal work night out with the usual banter and the usual silliness.

'See?' said Sarah. 'Nothing's changed!'

'And ain't it brilliant?' I replied.

Having been shortlisted for an award a few months previous (i.e., back when I had hair), I had been asked to provide the organisers with a photo of myself for them to display on the big screen when the nominees were announced. 'I know I wouldn't ordinarily be saying this,' I whispered to Keith during the ceremony, 'but I really really don't want to win tonight.'

'Photo?' he enquired, bang on the money.

'Exactly,' I confirmed. 'Nobody'll believe it's me.'

'Aw, give over, Lynchy,' he said, elbowing me. 'I'm still going to whoop at your name when it's read out, though.' And so he did, loudly and proudly, along with everyone else on our two tables, followed by a token 'bahh' when another nominee's name was announced as the award winner. I made a 'phew' gesture across the table and, this time at least, I meant it.

The following week saw the wedding of our good friends Sally and Ivan, at which I squeezed myself into some control underwear and stuck on some false eyelashes for a night of self-conscious dancing with the very unself-conscious Busby and her beau, Guy. Having just begun my daily five years' worth of Tamoxifen, the hormone-therapy drug designed to limit my body's ability to produce oestrogen, I was immediately suffering from the meno-pausal side effect of hot flushes, and spent much of the evening running to the loos to fan myself with my wig and run my pressure points under cold water. Busby and I had earlier devised a covert system of checking that my eye-lashes weren't being sweated off so when, as the night drew to a close, she began wildly waving her hands past her eyes on the dancefloor, I understood that she wasn't, in fact, doing her best impression of Mia Wallace at Jack Rabbit Slim's, but instead making me aware that my eyelashes were dangerously close to falling into a Hitler-style moustache.

The awards ceremony had completely tired me out and, given that it was taking a few days to get over, I volunteered to drive us to the wedding to save me turning narcoleptic over my champers and spare us all a costly cab journey home from Central London. On the way home, after dropping off Busby and Guy, P wanted to nip out of the car for a KFC. And so we pulled up on a double yellow line, blocking a driveway (proper bad-ass criminals that we are) and P jumped out for some late-night chicken.

While I waited I took off my wig, using the early-hours darkness as an excuse to be bald outside my flat. Suddenly a man appeared beside the car, gesturing through the window that he needed me to move back a bit so he could pull out. Forgetting myself, I opened the door to lean out and apologised, assuring him that I'd do it immediately – and then sat stunned as he moved a step closer towards me for a better view, looked amused, pointed a finger at my head and said, 'Ha. You've got no hair.'

And what do you say to that, eh? The man was right: I had no hair. Actually, if we're being pedantic, I did have a wee wispy bit of hair that was pushing its way through at that point, but I'm assuming it wasn't prominent enough to see in the dark. To him, I probably looked like the female version of the dying, mask-less Darth Vader at the end of *The Empire Strikes Back*. But still, hair or no hair, I didn't need him to remind me of my situation, thank you very much – particularly after having had such a lovely night.

'Some bloke just laughed at my bald head,' I said to P when he climbed back into the car.

'What? Who? Where is he?' snapped P, chucking the warm paper bag onto the back seat.

'He's gone now,' I said. 'He stepped towards me to look closer at it and everything.'

P got redder, his eyes widening in offended rage.

'But I didn't say anything back,' I concluded, puzzled.

I was upset about the rather odd exchange, of course, but for reasons other than the tactless tit saying what he did. I had missed an open-goal chance to use a retort I'd been practising since I first started losing my hair. I'm not proud to admit it, but I had been mentally preparing myself for such a perfect play-the-cancer-card moment for months. What I *should* have done outside KFC was stare back very seriously, giving him my best ill-person face and nodding sagely with slightly raised eyebrows before saying, 'That's because I've got *cancer.*' With careful, drawn-out emphasis on 'cancer'. Because, let's be honest, nothing stops people in their tracks like the word 'cancer'. But instead I frowned, looked at myself in the wing mirror (I don't know why; it wasn't like I had to check whether he was lying) and said, 'Er. Yeah.' Talk about a missed opportunity. I might have even got a bargain bucket out of the bastard.

CHAPTER 24

Escape to the country

December 2008

So then, sex. (Thought that'd get your attention.) And, more specifically, the wig on/wig off question. Oh come on, of course you've thought about it. I did nothing *but* think about it, once the wig-wearing reality had set in. Don't be fooled, here. It's not like P and I are having loads of sex at the moment. Cancer doesn't really allow much room/energy/desire for sex, and even simply knowing that The Bullshit is in your life kind of kills your mojo. But the wig-or-no-wig issue has been something I have, on occasion, had to call into question since my barnet did a bunk, and it's something I thought about once more the other night while watching *The Sopranos*.

Remember Svetlana, the one-legged, chain-smoking Russian home help? And remember the episode where she has sex with Tony on the sofa, while her prosthetic leg rests against the wall? Well, it got me thinking about what's worse: having sex with a woman without her prosthetic leg or without her wig? In the bigger picture, having no leg is obviously far worse than losing your hair through chemo but, thinking short-term, I'm tempted to conclude that most people would find a wigless partner more of a turn-off. Because, let's be honest, did you really spend your last shag looking at your other half's legs?

Fortunately P is only interested in wig-off mode. And for more than just sex. The moment we get home and our front door closes behind us, he's quick to whip off the syrup, despite the not-so-hot nature of what's underneath it. I'm still surprised by this. Not surprised that I'm married to a man so wonderful that he prefers his wife *au naturel*, but surprised that anyone can possibly prefer to see me the way that cancer intended. Since chemo ended, I've been busy convincing myself that the worst is over. Because, as much as I've trivialised it here, among the worst parts of The Bullshit for me has been – and continues to be – having to let other people see me like this.

I really wish I could have done a Kylie and fucked off to France for the duration of my treatment. Granted, with the paparazzi intrusion and all, she had more reason to turn recluse than I have, but that's not to say that I don't want to shut myself away any more than she did. And fair enough, I'm no Catherine Zeta-Jones in even my finest moments, but I *am* the kind of girl who only ever wants to be seen at her best, and not just looks-wise. So now that The Bullshit has washed its hands of my appearance, leaving me bald, bloated, blotchy and with a hefty dose of the blues, it takes hours of persuading – not to mention preening – myself before I'm game enough even to head out of the door.

And yes, the worst of the treatment is over (at least I hope it is). But, as P and I were forced to discover last week on our lovely break in the Lakes, no matter how far up the motorway you drive, and however little space you leave in your suitcase, cancer still finds a way to come with you.

*

With Sgt Pepper being spoilt at her grandparents' house, P and I took our first chance in months to escape for a few days on our own, away from the familiarity of the hospital and the chemist where we collected my prescriptions and the walls of our flat. Ordinarily, we're rather good at recognising our need for a break and buggering off somewhere different for the weekend, but cancer had, of course, put paid to that kind of stuff – and so we wanted to make this one count.

Now chemo was over we had a blissful interval before the next round of treatment, and we had assumed that this would be our opportunity to regain a bit of normal life; to enjoy a mini-break Lisa & P style, with gorgeous food, lovely wine, a stack of DVDs, country walks and loads of sex. And while we got the first three right, my dwindling energy levels saw to it that our walks – and our mattress gymnastics – were pitifully short.

But, of course, there was more to mine and P's frustration than our OAP-like bedroom antics (hell, the little nookie we managed was still a distinct improvement on the previous few months). Because escaping to the country unfortunately hadn't meant escaping from cancer. And by Friday, the tormenting thought of what was yet to come loomed large over the Lake District. It's like I told Mr Marbles: the Bullshit is as much a mental battle as it is a physical one. The medical world may know how to kill off a tumour, but it doesn't know how to rebuild the self-esteem that the tumour-busting treatment ruined in the process. So coming to terms with the magnitude of breast cancer, and the way it's changed your life, body and personality beyond recognition is an absurdly difficult task. And it's bound to overwhelm you every now and then, leaving you and your husband weeping into each other's dressing gowns on a Friday night in a hotel room in the hills, utterly unimpressed by the spectacular sunset that's competing for your attention.

After the gut-wrenching heartache of the previous night, the following evening P slept for two hours while I got myself back into the beautifying business of shaving my legs (all that talk of never whinging about doing it again was, of course, complete hooey) and preening the unusually straight pubes that had made their way back to my bikini line; all in an effort to appear ever so slightly more fanciable to my poor, sex-starved husband, who'd spent the past five months married to the uglier sister of George Dawes. And I'd forgotten what a palaver personal grooming was.

The menopause-inducing effects of Tamoxifen weren't doing much to help me in the looks department either, but I wondered whether my fall from femininity had less to do with my lack of oestrogen, and more to do with the simple fact that I was just out of practice when it came to being a girl? Cancer does not a woman make. Nor a man, for that matter. When you're in the throes of The Bullshit, you're neither man nor woman – you're a being. A being with one function: survive. There's just no space for anything else. Not shaving your legs or waxing your bikini line. Not spraying yourself with perfume or fake tan. Not choosing a pair of earrings in the morning, or making sure your bra matches your knickers. And especially not sex.

Later, with the grooming finished, we headed down for one of those amazing, drawn-out, drunken dinners where you talk for hours on end, completely ignoring the rest of the room. It was the first time we'd dared review our story so far. We talked about everything, from the day P grabbed hold of a lump in my left boob, to the horrors of my treatment. We talked about changing everyone's lives for ever as P made that impossible phone call to my dad with news of my diagnosis. The first time I looked down after my mastectomy to see the alien circle of skin where my nipple once was. The way none of us knew what to do, how to react or where to put ourselves when I fell so ill after the first chemo. The look on Jamie and Leanne's faces when they saw how the second chemo was affecting me. The first time P had to unblock the toilet of masses of my thick, blonde hair. The tantrum I threw at Tills when trying on my first wig. The helplessness of my father-in-law, and the chicken broth that he wished was a cure. The people who've been so fantastic and supportive, and those who've suddenly disappeared. And the way I used to refuse even to fetch a paper without first straightening my hair, and how ludicrous that seems now that my looks and self-confidence have sunk to their lowest.

It's only when you break it down like that, daringly pausing to remember the enormity of what you've been through, that you appreciate how completely bloody incredible you've been to endure everything you have. After six months like that, P and I ought to have been throwing ourselves off Scafell Pike, let alone crying into each other's arms before ordering room service.

Right back from That Day In June, I'd become used to having good weeks and bad weeks. And, in neat little units of one week, it was an emotional ride I could handle. But what was becoming increasingly testing was not knowing from one moment to the next whether I'd feel happy or upset or frustrated or angry or worried or tearful or what- ever else. It was a bit like having PMS all the time, only without the periods. And I was wary of it getting the better of me. There wasn't a lot I could do about it – with five years of Tamoxifen on the cards, it was something I was going to have to get used to – but I wrestled with the kind of person I feared I was becoming. I desperately didn't want to become one of those volatile, temperamental people that I'd always had such trouble with. Though Tamoxifen's other side-effects were hardly going to be a picnic – weak bones, weight gain, hot flushes and dryness in places you could do without being so desert-like – each of those things I could do something about. The mood-swing stuff, however, was something I had little means of reasoning with.

Marbles insisted that I shouldn't give myself such a hard time about something so difficult to control. The trouble was, my emotions just weren't that easy to separate. And so we concluded that it was okay to feel several conflicting things at one time without staring down the barrel of multiple personality disorder. It was okay to feel angry that I was spending so much time at the hospital, yet experience pangs of Stockholm Syndrome when my schedule of appointments decreased. It was okay to feel ecstatic that the worst part of my treatment was over, yet pissed off that there was still more to come. It was okay to appreciate the seriousness of my upcoming radiotherapy, yet find the YMCA position hilarious. It was okay to forget about having cancer for one wonderful minute, yet find myself angry when that moment passed. It was okay to want to spend a lifetime in the Lakes with nobody other than my husband, yet occasionally feel disappointed that we wouldn't have kids of our own to share it with. And it was okay to accept that my hormone therapy might make me a little unpredictable, yet still make an effort to keep my mood swings under wraps. All that said, if some arsewipe tried smirking at my slaphead again, I couldn't be held responsible for my actions, so help me, Tamoxifen.

CHAPTER 25

Wig out

I kinda like radiotherapy so far; it's been pretty cool. (Actually, it's been pretty scorching, but up to now the sunburn it's given me is no worse than I managed on honeymoon, when I singed the right side of my face with perfect precision while my iPod distracted me from the factor 30.) And yeah, the side-effects are going to build to the point where I'll probably come to regret that first sentence but, for the moment at least, radio is nothing I can't handle. Plus it's thrown up a very interesting discovery, but more of that later.

The treatment room where I'm having my radiotherapy is just down the corridor from the techno-tastic *Starship Enterprise* recording studio where I had my planning appointment, but looks much the same: space-age and hi-tech, but in a very 1980s way. It's silvery-grey with Commodore-esque computer screens and seemingly unattached keyboards in every corner, with bright strip lighting that occasionally dims to darkness. I was half expecting Five Star to walk in and re-film the 'System Addict' video. The radio girls on my shift (let's call them Pepsi & Shirlie) have clearly caught onto the 80s theme, too – four treatments in and so far their stereo has played Eurythmics,

New Order and the *Dirty Dancing* soundtrack. After shouting out numbers over the sound of the music and drawing on me with felt pen, they leave me alone in the room to let the radioactive waves do their work, all the while watching me on CCTV as I lie still, halfway through the YMCA, humming along to *Now That's What I Call The 1980s*.

When Pepsi & Shirlie come back, we fill our thirty-second conversation window with utter fluff, as they unstrap me from the leather bed (don't get excited) and move the machines back to a position where I won't headbutt them on the way out. I really like Pepsi & Shirlie. They're young, spritely, up for a giggle and constantly taking the piss out of each other. But it isn't like chemo, where you've got all day to natter with the nurses. With radio, you're not in there long enough for a proper chat, so instead you end up with scattered nuggets of random information about each other. What I know about Pepsi & Shirlie so far is that they like to ask about the weather, that Shirlie's going ice skating this week, that Pepsi prefers Gary but thinks Jason's been looking hot recently, and that they both use their later shifts as an excuse to go late-night shopping. And in return, they know that my kitten scratched the hell out of my left hand when I tried to wet-wipe her, that I'd bought and wrapped all my Christmas presents by mid-November, that I agree on the Gary/Jason front and that I've ditched my wig in favour of headscarves.

That's right, people. I'm scrapping the syrup. Or at least for the most part. You might think this an odd decision, but if I've learned one thing from having cancer it's that you can't always trust your opinions (hell, I've gone from animal-hater to cat-owner in the space of six months). It was all a bit of an accident, really, but by Monday it was clear that my wig needed washing (it only needs doing every three weeks, but then takes twenty-four to forty-eight hours to dry), so I had no choice but to go without it for the day. And, as I was pleasantly surprised to discover, I felt *far* less self-conscious wearing a headscarf than I ever had in my wig.

Actually I fibbed a bit back there. I did have a choice other than the headscarf: Wig 2 (aka Erika). I don't think I've ever communicated just how much I've **loathed** wearing a wig. (See, **loathed**. In bold and everything.) I hate that wig every bit as much as I hate the cancer that necessitated it. Aside from the fact that it's hugely unflattering, it's also itchy, annoying, I'm constantly aware of it, it embarrasses me and, frankly, in certain lights it's a bit on the ginger side. It's like carrying Geri Halliwell around on my head all day. And imagine having to prop her up on your bathroom window-sill every evening, where she'll freak you out when you get up in the night and be the first in-focus thing you see every morning. I've even stopped closing our bathroom door in the hope that Sgt Pepper might find it and claw it to pieces while I'm out.

Part of the reason I took the wig route in the first place was that I still wanted to feel desired. Early on in my wig-wearing days, I remember how chuffed I was when a man in the street appeared to check me out. Five months on, I fear I've even lost the desire to be desired, which is saying something given the fit boy on reception in radiotherapy. But oddly – when you consider the obvious, cancer-cards-on-the-table effects – there are vanity reasons behind the headscarf-wearing, too.

For one, I'm soon going to have short enough (or should that be long enough?) hair to be able to go without a wig or headscarf. And since I've had long locks all my life, I've got to learn to stop hiding behind my hair. (Translation: before I unveil my newborn-baby-chic hairdo, I need to get people used to seeing my moon face.) Then there's the paranoia it'll spare me: I'd rather people came to the cancer conclusion after thinking, 'That girl's wearing a headscarf' than, 'Do you reckon that's a wig?'

So I'm giving up the ghost (well, except for special occasions, perhaps: weddings, parties, posh restaurants, the football . . .). I'm coming out of the cancer closet. And, to paraphrase George Michael, the game that I'm giving away just isn't worth playing. Freedom!

*

Over Christmas dinner one year, Nan pointed to the scarf I was using as a headband and noted, 'That thing makes you look like a gypsy.' She wasn't one to mince her words, was Nan, but despite most of the things she said to me being unnecessarily flattering, this comment has stayed with me ever since. And, whether or not I admitted it at the time, it was also the reason I chose the wig route rather than the headscarf one.

For a while, it was the right thing to do. When it comes to The Bullshit, you've got to accept pretty early on that the best way to play it is to do whatever feels right at the time – and sod any consequences or previously rigid opinions you may have held. The beauty is, at least, that nobody's going to question you on it. Hate animals but want a cat? Go for it, let's call the RSPCA. Ask for salmon for dinner but then gag at the smell from the kitchen? No problem, there's pasta in the cupboard. Insist on spending £400 on wigs then ditch the lot? Whatever makes you happy. And so, within five months, I'd gone from insisting on disguising my cancer from the world with wigs, eyebrow pencils and fake tan, to completely giving up the ghost with headscarves and a take-me-as-you-find-me attitude. Aside from that, though, it made radiotherapy easier to negotiate. The daily routine of a morning hospital visit on which I had to lie in the same uncomfortable position wasn't exactly conducive to wig-wearing, and with my cancer-specialist hospital being the only place I was ever seen in public, I was hardly doing a wonderful impression of a healthy average Joe anyway.

Pitiful as it was when compared to the chemo-ills, the burn-like pain that came with radiotherapy was beginning to wind me up as much as the monotonous routine. I'd somehow managed to get away with its annoying effects after the first week but, after the second, the radio-targeted cross-section of my body had become burned, painful, itchy and achy. It was starting to give my left arm jip, too, to the point where my fingers repeatedly swelled up like one of those giant foam hands you get at the baseball or in the audience on *Gladiators*. And so, with primary lymphoedema seemingly causing the trouble, I was referred to the lymphoedema clinic, where they fitted me for the best, hi-tech, swelling-solving device that contemporary medical science has to offer: a stretchy glove. It wasn't even a nice-looking glove, either. It was cut-off-your-circulation tight, skin coloured (well, it is if you're Nancy Dell'Olio) and fingerless, with messy-looking seams on the outside. But even that wasn't credibility-destroying enough for the nurses in the clinic, who also taught me some daily physio-therapy exercises that were basically tantamount to doing the 'Birdie Song'. (Add that to the 'YMCA' and I'm prac-tically ready to audition for a place in The Nolans.)

The absurdity didn't stop there. There was the sunburnt skin, too. Actually, that I had accounted for, but not the swelling. Overnight, it seemed, my left boob had grown a cup size bigger than my right, and my saline implant was hardening with every treatment. It was the first side-effect I'd felt in my breast since the mastectomy, and it brought home to me yet again how I kept forgetting the still-unfathomable fact that all of this began with a tumour in my boob. My lovely boob. One of the few parts of my body that I'd always said I wouldn't change (just like I always said that alopecia was among my biggest fears – seems you don't have to be careful what you wish for; more what you're afraid of). But that was six months ago – now it had become a huge, round lump of hardened, red Play-Doh, without even the crowning glory of a nipple.

My boob had only ever had what I consider a modest number of public outings and a tiny part of me wished that I'd let it have its day – a page-three photo shoot, some topless sunbathing, or a cheeky chavvy flash on someone's shoulders in the crowd of an Oasis gig. But that number wouldn't be increasing now, and not just because there was a ring on my finger. I wondered what I'd do in the future sex-wise if I weren't married. I was – and still am – intrigued to know what single, Bullshit-befallen women do when they're recovered and having fun and ready to get back on the horse? Because how do you broach the subject? The I've-had-breast-cancer line is something of a turn-off, no? Or is it the ultimate test of a man, to see whether or not he's bothered by it? Does it make you a bra-on girl for evermore? Should you even mention it beforehand, or just crack on and see whether he notices?

At the current stage of my reconstruction, there was no hiding the fact. With a Toffee Penny for a left nipple, my bust was hardly the stuff that wet dreams are made of. And, as I discovered in my second week of radiotherapy – when, due to the pre-Christmas schedule of shifts, Pepsi & Shirlie were joined by two male nurses in the treatment room and became Bucks Fizz – P was no longer the only bloke who had to look me in the nipple and keep a straight face. So far, all but two of the medical professionals I'd seen had been women, and the male ones had been considerably older than me. But now, all of a sudden, there were two lads my age charged with the task of radiating my bust (and neck and shoulder and armpit, but I was less bothered about those bits), and I couldn't help but wonder what they thought of me and my bizarre bosom.

Not that the opinion of other men should matter, of course. Luckily, all I really needed to concern myself with was whether or not P could stand the sight of a naked new-me, and experience suggested that it wasn't going to be a problem. But that didn't stop me worrying about it. And so one day, I decided to test the water with the radio boys, and do my best to judge whether I completely grossed them out.

'You're a bit glammed up for radio, aren't you?' asked P.

'Good, I'm glad you noticed,' I answered, trying to find a pair of earrings to match my most glamorous headscarf.

'Yeah, but why?'

'It's an experiment,' I said. 'There's a couple of lads my age doing my radio this week and I need to know whether they're repulsed by me.'

P rolled his eyes. After two years of marriage, he knew better than to question another of my typically trivial trials that, more often than not, would be more at home in a Scooby Doo cartoon than real life.

'Well, I just hope it's got nothing to do with the boy on reception, is all,' he continued, shooting me an accusatory look. 'I read on your blog that you fancy him.'

'Oh, God, hardly,' I retorted. 'Besides, giving him a wink every day is just a bit of fun to liven up the monotony. You'll be coming next week, anyway, and you can see for yourself that he's no P Lynch.'

'Yeah, whatever,' he said. 'But if the boot was on the other foot . . .'

'I know, I know,' I admitted. 'Still, nobody's really going to be lusting after your cancer-patient wife, are they?'

And so into the radiotherapy floor I strutted, all head-scarf, heels and lip gloss, indulging in a morning mini-flirt with the boy on reception, and extending it a bit further down the corridor to try my luck in the treatment room, too. Radio Boy 1 was Play-Doh in my hands: one highly unoriginal comment about being topless in a dark room, and we were bang into the banter. Radio Boy 2 proved harder to break. I threw everything at it, from the local drinking holes to their Christmas-party scandal, but nothing doing. And just when I gave up and resorted to my usual inane gossip-column chatter – this time about Rihanna, how I was making her my hair muse and how I thought it a pity that she and Chris Brown clearly weren't right for each other when they look so cute together in photos – I finally got my answer. Radio Boy 2 was, indeed, appalled by the sight of my tits. But it turned out that not even Rihanna was his thing – he much preferred her fella. So I was happy to admit defeat on those grounds. And anyway, much like my status quo on the nipple front, one out of two wasn't bad.

CHAPTER 26

And never brought to mind

I'll make no bones about it: I'm struggling to deal with The Bullshit as much now as I was mid-chemo. I may have got my head around the physical effects and the things I need to do in response to them (nothing, mostly – radio is making me more exhausted by the day), but the myriad mental matters are tying me in knots.

Mid-sprout during my Christmas dinner, I found myself *this* close to throwing down my knife and fork, chucking my plate at the wall (like they do in the soaps) and screaming 'what the hell are we doing?' at P and my folks. In that moment, I simply could not believe that, regardless of what had happened this year, there we were, eating turkey and wearing paper hats as though it were a perfectly average 25 December. (My suspicion that a paper hat would substitute nicely for a headscarf was quickly quashed – from the shoulders up, I looked like a novelty eggcup.) The simple act of 'getting on with it' sometimes seems so preposterous in light of having been diagnosed with breast cancer, and every now and then I find myself irrationally angry with the rest of the world for going about its business as normal. EVERYTHING has changed for me, so why is everyone else carrying on as though nothing has happened?

Part of me wants to have a word with myself. 'For fuck's sake, you've got cancer. So what? Get over it.' And admittedly, most of the time (this blog excepted) I'm pretty flippant about having breast cancer – in public at least – preferring to make glib jokes, trivialise it and avoid giving it the grim respect it craves by smiling my way through as much as possible. But the other half of me appreciates – and is completely panicked by – the weight of this shitty episode, and wants to do something equally absurd in response. I sometimes feel like I'm perched on top of a volcano, and that at some point I'm going to do a Cameron Frye and completely flip out. I think it'd be only fair. Something as momentous as breast cancer in your twenties deserves a freak-out as big as Jacko's skin-colour-change or Britney's head-shave (insert obvious joke here). Drug dependency is out – I've had enough drugs to last me a lifetime this past few months – and I dare say I've already gone down the Elvis-inspired weight-gain route (Operation Elfin begins in earnest tomorrow). So maybe now's the time to get the tattoo, then?

I do have a few New Year resolutions, though, and one of them is that next year, I'd like *Alright Tit* to go from being about living with The Bullshit to being about wrestling my way out of it. I'm done with breast cancer and what it's done to me, the way it's made me look, the issues it's made me confront, the effect it's had on my life and the lives of my family and friends. Never before have I needed a new start as much as I do now. From this point on, *Alright Tit* is about getting *over* breast cancer, rather than getting *through* it.

That said, it's a tricky balance to negotiate. I don't want to be defined by having had breast cancer, but at the same time it *is* a pretty fucking big deal, so I *do* want people to know that I got through it. And while we're at it, I'd like a reward for getting through it, too. When people climb Everest or sprint quickly or jump high or give a brilliant movie performance, they get something in return. Well, this is my Everest, dammit, and if I have to make my own medal from tin foil and leftover Christmas ribbon, so be it. I just can't get my head around the fact that you can go through all of this and be expected to carry on again as normal, with nothing to show for your experience. (And yes, that *was* a Louboutins hint.)

*

Given that this was the first Christmas since Grandad died, the celebrations were always going to be somewhat muted, and so I guess if ever there was a festive period to waste on cancer, this was it. Charged with the responsibility of doing Christmas dinner for the first time in our lives, P and I entered into the spirit by flapping like pre-slaughter turkeys and buying more trimmings than it was possible to squeeze into our flat – because, of course, no Christmas would be complete without plum-pudding mini muffins, cinnamon-scented candles and three types of cranberry sauce.

Though Christmas day itself proved a quiet feast for four (P, me, Mum and Dad), I did manage to squeeze in a couple of parties over the season. With work dos and late-night pub visits out of the question thanks to my increasing tiredness, I was forced into more home-based shindigs (i.e., the ones where I'd have a sofa or bed to collapse onto when necessary). So it was lucky, then, that Tills and Si agreed to host one of their legendary house parties with the help of my legendary (if I do say so myself) party playlist. And, wow. What a release. Wearing heels for the first time in too long and with no radiotherapy appointment the following day, I danced as long as I was able, to a soundtrack I'd purposely amended to allow myself a breather between each of my favourite, must-dance-to tracks.

While throwing some shapes with my mate (and Everybody's Favourite Dance Partner) Martin to 'Common People', I looked across to the sofa to find P grinning up at me with what my family now refer to as 'those eyes': the same gaze they witnessed as we exchanged vows at our wedding. I shuffled over in his direction, giving him a curious 'what are you thinking?' look. 'Later,' he mouthed, shaking his head and gesturing for me to head back to the routine I shared with Martin.

'What was that all about?' I asked P on the way home.

'That was brilliant,' he said enthusiastically. 'Brilliant. You were dancing around like a lunatic.'

'Ha, cheers!' I laughed.

'I don't mean it like *that*, nobhead,' P continued. 'It was brilliant because I just felt total joy when I looked at you.'

'Oh, babe,' I said, linking my arm with his. 'That's lovely. Me too.'

'It's just so long since I've seen that,' he said, misty eyed. 'It was like looking at a glimpse of the past that was taken away from us.'

I nodded.

'But most importantly,' he continued, rather profoundly, 'I was getting a first glimpse of our wonderful future, too.'

P was right. With the new year came a glimmer of hope that 2009 couldn't possibly be as much of a git as its predecessor and, as I'd said on my blog, I was determined for the next few months to be about getting *over* cancer – not scrapping my way through it. But with every new year comes a hangover, and mine wasn't just the treatment I was yet to have, but also coming to terms with what had happened. Getting over cancer wasn't something I was going to be able to do on my own – just as the cancerous burden in my breast needed help in being removed, so did the equally cancerous burden in my mind. And my fear of what sort of life I'd have once I'd finished treatment weighed heavily on me.

My initial reason for going to therapy was that I wanted help moving on to a life in which cancer would be a mere detail, but what I also wanted was to figure out what kind of life that might be. After such a monumental bump in the road, what could possibly come next? At least that's what I thought I was worried about. And I'd have gone on thinking that was the problem, had I not met Mr Marbles.

Marbles is the Columbo of therapy. He'd lead me off in one direction, and just when I thought I'd spewed forth everything I had to offer, he'd play the 'just one more thing' card and yank out the real issue quicker than you can say trenchcoat (or corduroy slacks). So there I was in session three, having a guilt-free whinge about not knowing what to do next when he suddenly turned school careers advisor on me and asked where I'd like to be in six months, a year, two years and five years. I talked about the fun I was going to have with P and Tills and Si at Glastonbury, the pubs I was looking forward to meeting my mates in, the funky haircut I wanted, the work I was anxious to get back into, the holidays I was going to plan, the house I wanted to buy, the book I intended to write and the butterfly-like change from being the girl who has cancer into the girl who *beat* cancer. Or, better yet, just *the girl*. (Is it still okay to call yourself a girl when you're thirty?)

And there it was. Case closed. My concern wasn't my ability to make a life plan (that exercise was proof enough that my arrangement-making skills are as good as ever), but that cancer forces might cut short the plans I did make. By the end of my quick-fire life-planning with Marbles, I'd burst into tears.

'Forget all that,' I told him. 'In five years, I just want to still be here.'

And therein lies the problem with trying so hard to move on. You can't just neatly decide to do it when you dance in heels for the first time, or when a new year comes along to box things off so seemingly tidily. It just doesn't work like that. Because there's so much more to deal with than just the diagnosis and treatment and getting yourself well again.

As soon as you're diagnosed, everyone talks about your chance of survival. And, as though the diagnosis weren't frightening enough, the five- and ten-year survival rates make for pretty grim reading. (Despite the size and spread of my cancer, my number was 'about 70 per cent', thanks to my age and the most kick-ass cancer treatment the NHS can offer.) But then the whirlwind of drugs and hospital visits begins, and everyone suddenly stops talking about your chance of survival, opting instead for the can-do attitude of *when* rather than *if.* And you get swept along with it. But once the chemo horrors had come to an end, and I found myself squinting in the face of the disco lights at the end of the tunnel, I was suddenly back to worrying about that 30 per cent-ish chance of not being around to stick a middle finger up to the statistics.

I don't often get angry. I like to think I'm pretty *que sera sera* (if you brush aside refereeing decisions, misplaced apostrophes and the BBC's insistence on wheeling out Heather Small to sing 'Search For The Hero' at sporting ceremonies). But the fact that I was having to confront how long I had left at the age of twenty-nine was a pretty fucking difficult pill to swallow. It was unfair and it was painful – and not just for me. So, for those very reasons, I did my darndest to avoid talking about it. But, as Marbles reminded me, I had always spoken of breast cancer as an equal battle of body and mind. I'd blogged about my bowel movements and my missing nipple, so why not my mortality?

'So why is it that you won't blog about your fears of death?' he asked, crosslegged and tapping on his notebook with a Biro.

'Well, because I'm British,' I retorted. 'And we just don't talk about death, do we?'

Death is the ultimate unmentionable. Regardless of the situation, it tends to be the elephant in the room. It's what you immediately think of upon being told you have cancer (well, with me it was hair first, death second). And yet, as soon as the diagnosis is done with, nobody mentions it again. I hadn't spoken or blogged about death previously because I didn't want to upset my family.

But now, mid-therapy and suddenly more capable of telling people what I felt, I began to hope that some kind of relief would come from the fact that I was finally prepared to talk – nay, blog – about it. 'To bring it down to crude basics,' I wrote, 'if I die, I die – I'd not have to deal with it any more than that. Which is why it's much more difficult for my family and friends to have to think about. And why, for me at least, it's harder to consider the death of someone I love than it is to consider dying myself. But if that's the case, so be it. There's not a damn thing I can do about it, other than to keep doing what I'm doing. What will be, will be.'

I had often thought that having cancer felt a bit like experiencing all the best bits of dying, without me actually having to pop my clogs. ('The best bits of dying' . . . sheesh, I don't half have a dark sense of humour.) And, always keen to find a bright side to these things, I reckoned that made me lucky. I'd smelled the flowers at my own funeral. When someone dies, they don't always get to know how loved they were. But I had been left in no doubt. I'd been told 'I love you' more often than I ever expected to hear it. It still didn't make me pleased that I got cancer, mind, but without it I wouldn't have appreciated the staggering volume of terrific people around me. It's not often you get to look back on your life (so far) in this way. And while on one hand the realisation of how good I'd got it meant that I had more to lose, on the other hand it gave me so much more to fight for. So when I put it in terms of the happy, fulfilled life I'd led even before I'd hit thirty, the issue of 'the end' somehow seemed a little less scary.

Not that I plan on letting the five-year (hell, even fifty-year) survival stats get in my way. There was – and still remains – a lot left on my to-do list. I've got to see Derby County win the Premiership, for one. And, in the mean-time, I had a festival to get drunk at, a book to write, a flat to decorate, a husband to grow old with and a blonde wig ready and waiting for my octogenarian years. Old-fashioned it may be, but I dare say it'll look a heck of a lot more hip than a blue rinse.

CHAPTER 27

Rehab

January 2009

Well, I don't know about you, Winehouse, but I say yes, yes, yes. Step aside, Lohan. Out of the way, Moss. Your time is up, Williams. Search my bag and save me a room at The Priory; I'm on a one-way ticket to self-improvement.

Like I said last year, 2009 is the year of Sorting Shit Out. Seriously, check the Chinese zodiac. (Do you like how I said 'last year' back then? See, it's all just a bad memory.) This is the year when I'll be able to once again pick up a hairdryer, go bra shopping, have more sex, pay attention to my bikini line, get off my steroid-swelled arse and generally execute a Houdini-like escape from the evil grip of The Bullshit. Ta-dah!

Right now, I don't look great. Actually that's somewhat generous. I look like the long-lost sister of Tweedledum and Tweedledee. And it's time to do something about it. I appreciate that it'll take a fair bit of doing, which is why I intend to kick off early, before the final whistle of my surgery and the end of my active treatment. I'm realistic about the timeframe, too – hell, I've not just got hair to grow, but weight to shift, a left tit to transform, eyelashes to sprout and eyebrows to fill. So the plan is this: screw my twenties, I'm writing them off. Instead, I'm going to make damn sure I look super-hot in preparation for my thirties, just in time to flaunt the New Me at my Super Sweet 30th. (From its conception with Busby on my sofa, I've taken the idea a step further and have decided to turn it into a charity fundraiser for Breast Cancer Care. Well, you know how I like a project.)

But back to Operation Elfin. The issue here is that cancer is forcing me into an image change. Just as bouncing back to the life I had pre-Bullshit is unrealistic, so is the thought that I'll have my long blonde locks back the moment I'm brave enough to whip off my headscarf. Right now, the trouble is less length, more coverage. And since Wikipedia tells me that human hair grows at a rate of 0.4mm per day, I reckon the most I'm looking at is a Posh-Spice-style pixie crop by the time I hit Glastonbury. But of course, if I'm going to carry off hair like Rihanna/ Gwyneth/Posh, I'm going to need the frame to suit it. So as well as the hair-spurt mission, I'm also on a shrink-down health-kick to shift the 16lbs (shock! horror!) that cancer so kindly gifted me. (My fitness DVD will be in the shops next Christmas.)

I'm thinking of the unwanted bulk as a bit like baby weight, but without actually having had to squeeze one out. And, if you think about it, it's not all that far off, really: several months of suffering, the removal of a funny-shaped lump from my body, the sleepless nights, even the mothering – albeit kitten rather than baby. Still, baby weight/cancer weight, potato/potahtoe – whatever you want to call it, it's on the way out.

Health-wise I'm still a long way off jogging round the park (hell, even jogging to the loo). Radiotherapy continues to take its toll, and the exhaustion is reminding me of the time at uni when I had one too many late nights, snogged one too many smelly boys and ended up with glandular fever. But as much as it's kicking me up the arse when I'm not there, I don't half love having somewhere to go every day, and a brilliant bunch of people to see it through with. It's like going into the office – I chirp a cheery hello to the (still fit) boy on reception, say 'good morning' to the other eleven-o'clock regulars in the waiting room, then enjoy a bit of banter with the radio staff.

For the last couple of weeks, it's been my favourite lass and lad in the radio room (from Pepsi & Shirlie to Bucks Fizz, and now Dollar). I love Dollar (seriously, this is getting daft). They always let me in on the department in-jokes and the three of us have a right good giggle every morning (plus I think I've gained a few favouritism points after slipping them some golden gossip nuggets from my LA-reporter pal Ant). I've only got nine treatments left, and I'm going to miss the arses off those two when I finish. Do you think it's acceptable to befriend them on Facebook? Or is the cupcake-baking option a better display of gratitude?

*

When I posted a not-far-past-bald photo of myself online, I was overwhelmed with messages.

'This is *exactly* the right thing to do,' assured Tills.

'I'm a bit scared to tell you this in light of you having banned this word,' said Weeza, 'but that's a brave thing you've done.'

But the truth, I fear, was that uploading the photo was done more out of cowardice than bravery.

It began with a new-year get-together at our place. With Ant home from Los Angeles for the holidays, we invited the old gang – Tills, Si, Polly, Martin – round to the flat for a festive curry and cava session. It was the first time Ant had seen me since my trip to LA in the time between finding my lump and discovering what kind of havoc the lump was capable of causing.

'Oh, Mac!' she exclaimed as I opened my front door. 'You still look exactly like you!'

'I bloody hope not,' I said. 'I don't particularly *want* to look like this!'

'Oh fuck off,' she answered, thrusting a bottle of cava into my hand. 'You're gorgeous. End of.'

Now, I adore Ant, and I adore her even more for complimenting me on the way I looked when I was wearing a dodgy wig (this being a special circumstance, I left the headscarf in a drawer) and a dress that was a couple of sizes too small. But Ant, on this occasion, was wrong. I didn't look gorgeous. I looked horrendous. But I didn't realise quite how horrendous I looked until Ant uploaded the photos of her trip onto Facebook.

'Antonia tagged a photo of you,' said the email.

'Oh shit,' I thought, clicking on the link. 'This can't be good.'

June 2008 to January 2009 had been a mostly photo-free zone; only at Jamie and Leanne's wedding did I accept that a camera would be pointing in my direction and, since that was after a spray-tan and professionally applied make-up, I was prepared to let it go.

'You've GOT to delete that photo,' I pleaded with Ant in an email immediately after un-tagging myself. 'That photo isn't of me. That photo is of a fat lass in a wig. And I DO NOT want people to see me that way.'

I'm not one for *ever* having cross words with my friends, and I knew that Ant would be surprised by my unusually angry tone. It wasn't cool, kicking up a fuss in that way, and after pressing send I instantly felt bad for writing such a narky email. But in truth, I was seething.

This was supposed to be my fresh start; the beginning of not just a new year, but a new life, too. But on that day, crying into my laptop at the sight of what The Bullshit had done to me, it couldn't have felt further from that. There I was, sobbing at a photograph of myself effectively in disguise, when what lay underneath it was just as unpleasant. And so, figuring that it was time to slowly come out of hiding my appearance, I took the first photo of myself *sans* wig, posted it online and sent it to Ant with an apology.

My cancer disguise wasn't without its uses, mind you. The following week, towards the end of radiotherapy, with my session having overrun by about, ooh, three weeks, I ran (okay, walked quickly) back to the car to find a traffic warden standing over it, tapping away on his ticket machine, licking his lips and circling my Astra like a hungry bird of prey. You know how parking attendants always tell you they've already started making out your ticket and can't possibly stop, even though you're back now? Well, THEY LIE. Because this dude stopped and scarpered. And I swear it was because of my headscarf.

It wasn't the first time that my headscarf got me preferential treatment. Earlier that morning, in the packed radiotherapy waiting room, a woman gave up her chair for me. 'Oh here, love,' she smiled. 'You have this seat – I'm not a patient.' And the previous week, on my way back from the hospital in a minor traffic jam on Chelsea Embankment, I managed to silence a very shouty, road-raged woman who was shrieking abuse at anyone in her path from the window of her MX5, and refusing to let anyone in despite them blocking up the adjacent lane. When our cars aligned, with windows rolled down, I looked calmly in her direction and said, 'Just what have *you* got to

214

moan about, lady?' She had nothing to say. And, by 'eck, it felt good.

Grateful as I was for such minor cancer upsides, I started to wonder whether there was a moral question here. While I was sure that nobody would deny a cancer patient taking advantage of some assistance whenever they could, at what point did accepting assistance become milking it? When it came to playing the cancer card, what were the rules? It isn't exclusively a cancer game, of course. There's a range of suits in this deck: cancer, health, age, sex . . . And it's perfectly acceptable, is it not, to play the pregnancy card – whether for a seat on the tube or a free upgrade on the train. So, by that token, is the cancer excuse fair game? (I'll see your stomach cramps and raise you a bald head.)

There's no point giving you my poker face here – breast cancer was an excuse I had been known to use on occasion. But not half as much as I could have done, or even as much as I'd like to have done. I'm a long way off getting comfy on the moral high ground. Because while I believe that the cancer card should be reserved only for mischief purposes on special occasions, like a pair of red heels you keep for big nights out, I sure as eggs is eggs wouldn't begrudge anyone using it whenever they bloody well wanted.

When driving to my daily appointments, I often wondered what I'd do if I got pulled over for speeding. There was every chance I would, as well, given the insufficient time I left myself to get to the hospital every morning (who am I kidding – the insufficient time I leave myself to get *anywhere*). And there was no doubt about it – with no cleavage card at my disposal, hell yeah, I'd have dug deep for the cancer cop-out. And I'd be willing to wager that you'd do the same.

The thing was, in my second calendar year of cancer, I reckoned I'd paid my dues. I'd served my time, done the stretch of torturous treatment and got The Bullshit on my permanent record. I'd earned it – that card was mine to play. Cancer doesn't exactly come with benefits. Your consultant doesn't set the ball rolling with, 'Well, I'm afraid you've got cancer. But hey, at least the Sainsbury's delivery man will carry your groceries through to the kitchen.'

P was never so quick to play the cancer card. Not that he hadn't considered it, mind. One day he came home from work with a bee in his bonnet about a colleague who'd pissed him off all day with her vocal, reasonless whinging. 'What about?' I enquired.

'Oh, I dunno. The weather or her waistline or a bad hair day or something. All I wanted to do was grab her by the neck and say, "Shut the fuck up, woman. Do you know what I've been going through?"'

But he didn't. Because P is better than that. In fact, very few people in his office even knew that he was nursing his wife through breast cancer. It was something he kept as quiet as he could in his professional life, wishing simultaneously to avoid anyone's pity and to continue in his work as he always would have done.

When something like cancer muscles in on your life, you don't half find yourself low on patience for other people's dubious gripes. So I'd even go so far as to say that I think it's okay for someone to play the cancer card on your behalf. (Within reason, like – I don't want you to go missing a deadline tomorrow and blaming it on me.)

Having cancelled two holidays and countless other days out last year because of me, my folks booked themselves a well-deserved, pre-Christmas long weekend in New York. At check-in, they could see that the flight had been overbooked and the attendant was busy bumping people off the plane.

'What will we do if they try to stop us getting on?' asked Mum.

'That woman will hear *exactly* what kind of year I've had,' replied my old man. And good on him.

CHAPTER 28

To the end

One mastectomy, five months of chemotherapy, six weeks of radiotherapy, and I'm done. My active cancer treatment (if you don't count the last bit of surgery and five years of Tamoxifen) is over. Finished. And I swear I just saw a tumbleweed roll past my bedroom window.

The other day, I was sitting on the sofa with Mum, reading the comments that people have left on my blog.

'I can't believe all this has happened,' she said.

'I know, it's ace, right? All these people I've never met being so nice to me – I don't know what to do with it,' I replied.

Mum looked puzzled. 'Well, yes, that is lovely, but I didn't mean that,' she explained. 'I meant all of this. Breast cancer. I can't believe it's happened to you.'

As it goes, neither can I. It's almost eight months since my diagnosis, seven months since my mastectomy, six months since chemo began and six weeks since my first radiotherapy session. Eight whole months of talking and worrying and crying and obsessing and blogging about cancer, and I'm not sure whether I should be deliriously happy that it's over or really fucking angry that it happened in the first place. I'm furiously flitting between hyperactive, party-seeking emancipation and disbelieving, panic-stricken remembrance of the whole hideous ordeal. But mostly I'm numb. Weepy and exhausted and numb.

Has the reality of having breast cancer really only just hit me? It feels like I've been thrown straight back into that same black hole I found myself lost in at the beginning, in that awful, helpless time between diagnosis and treatment when there's nothing to do but read frightening things on the internet and try to convince yourself that you're not going to die. Then, on the eve of my final treatment, I had a panic attack. At least I think I did. I'm not certain I've had one before. But I had that same gut-wrenching, pulse-racing, heart-sinking, colour-draining, future-fearing feeling I had back in June.

I want this to be an uplifting story. I want to pick myself up, dust myself down and get on with whatever it is I've got to get on with now. So does everyone around me – whatever they say, I'm sure I can sense their frustration that I'm not quite well enough (physically or mentally) to bounce back into life as we all knew it. And fair enough – while I've talked and worried and cried and obsessed and written about The Bullshit for almost eight months, they're the ones who've had to hear it all. They're as sick of it as I am. They must feel like they're on the receiving end of a proud parent's single topic of conversation. But I also want this to be an honest story. And the honest truth is this: at the end of treatment there's as much to mourn as there is to celebrate.

There's a terrific Macmillan-run online cancer support community that I discovered recently, called *What Now?* And, to the untrained, unaffected-by-cancer ear, that's just a simple, snappy, easy-to-remember title. But, to anyone who's walked in my size sevens (spot the Louboutins hint), calling a cancer support community *What Now?* is actually a stroke of brilliant, heart-of-the-truth genius.

'Tills? What the . . .?'

'Happy end of treatment day!' she squealed, hoisting a giant, ribboned bottle of cava in the air as I walked towards my radiotherapy treatment room for the final time.

'You sneaky bugger,' I said, grabbing her for a hug. 'Who told you where to come?'

'Well, P was in on it,' she said. 'He gave me the directions and times and all that. Oh, and I spotted the fit boy on reception, by the way.'

'Ha, yeah. I thought P had been quiet,' I said, taking a seat beside her in the waiting room, and placing the assorted cupcakes I'd baked for the staff on the floor in front of my feet. 'Actually, I wondered why he hadn't volunteered to come himself today, but I guess I can let him off now, eh?'

'Absolutely,' asserted Tills. 'Anyway, I didn't want you going straight home on your own after this, so I'm taking you out for lunch instead.'

'You are a *wonderful* mate, Tillface,' I said, pinching her knee.

As only a close friend can, Tills knew without me even having to mention it that my final day of radiotherapy had the potential to be a rather emotional one. Finally at the end of my meticulously choreographed treatment routine and being released from capture, she knew as well as I did that I wouldn't quite know where to put myself once I didn't have a hospital-issued timetable telling me where to go next. Getting out of the habit of planning ahead had been the first hurdle for me to negotiate after my diagnosis – despite it going against every grain of my being, the only way to keep myself sane was to bow to the cliché and take every day as it came. Which was precisely what I'd been doing for seven months – but now, I had to switch it off again and find a route back to my old way of life. And it wasn't quite as easy as it sounded.

'Are you going to be okay for the rest of the day?' asked a concerned Tills after we left the Yo! Sushi in which I'd cried over my tempura.

'I'll be fine,' I said. 'I'm sorry today wasn't more celebratory, especially after you made all this effort.'

'Lady,' said Tills with an arm around my shoulder, 'I think we know by now that The Bullshit doesn't let us celebrate when we want to. But our time will come. You know that, right?'

'I know, I know,' I said. 'And hey, in the meantime I've got a magnum of cava to work my way through and there's a Krispy Kreme stall across the road with my name on it.'

'That's my girl,' chirped Tills, leading me back towards the car park.

Having finished radiotherapy on a Monday (as if to prove that cancer treatment never ends neatly), the remainder of the week was just as unsettling. And, as it turned out, my pre-finale panic attack wasn't to be my last. I had always assumed that panic attacks were like fits: palpitations, tunnel vision, dizziness, passing out and calling a doctor. Much like cancer, I had filed them under It'll Never Happen To Me and got on with my life. But throughout the week it became clear that they were muscling in on things, too; these unpleasant, terrifying, uncontrollable moments that would overwhelm me, take my breath, make me shiver and reduce me to dizzy tears in the rare times that I wasn't keeping myself busy.

The busy thing was key. Pre-Bullshit, I used to love doing nothing. I'd spend many a contented hour lying on my back, happy with my thoughts. I once lived on my own, too, and loved every second. I was always good in my own company, doing sod all. But suddenly, I was never doing nothing, and never on my own (at the risk of sounding like Liz Jones, I consider Sgt Pepper company). Even when I was silent, my mind would be plugging away at something or other. Just as there's always a song in my head, at that point there was always a job to be done, an email to be sent, a Facebook status to update, a tweet to post, a list to write . . . for an inherently lazy lass, I was doing a damn good job of keeping myself busy. And it was a state I was keen to keep myself in, purely because I couldn't afford *not* to be busy. Because that was when the panic attacks would come.

The problem, of course, was that the more I sat on the shit stuff by staying distracted, the more it would come back to bite me on the ass. The anxiety remained, bubbling under the surface, forcing its way out like angry steam from a boiling pan in 101 unhelpful 'what ifs'. What if the cancer came back? What if the treatment hadn't worked? What if there was another tumour I didn't know about? What if there were cancer cells I wasn't aware of? What if I only had a short time left? Which was how I ended up making an idiot of myself at the hospital later that week.

The Friday following the end of my radiotherapy had been a red X on my calendar for months: the day on which the end of my active treatment would be neatly bookended with a final visit to the Curly Professor's Glamorous Assistant. In my wildest dreams (and I'm just the kind of idiot who believes their wildest dreams), I was going to walk out of that appointment having heard a joyous clasp of hands and a sentence that began, 'Well, your treatment was a resounding success . . .' and perhaps even the word 'remission'. Idiot indeed. Instead, the information I was left with proved a sledgehammer of a reminder of how serious my diagnosis was.

'So, can we say I'm in remission now?' I asked Glamorous Assistant, while tearing holes in a tissue with one hand and gripping onto P with the other (he'd had holes torn into him that morning with the kind of narky, fret-induced nagging that he used to endure each Chemo Friday).

'No no no, not yet,' she said, as though I'd asked whether she might be able to create a French plait from my cropped locks. 'The problem with the word remission is that it applies to a time when treatment has ended, and since you'll be taking Tamoxifen for five years, your active treatment won't have finished until you've stopped taking that.'

'Great,' I spat, trying to force back my tears with attitude. 'I just thought you'd be telling me I was in remission today.'

'I'm sorry; I can't yet,' she said, demonstrably sympathetic to my disappointment. 'The discourse around cancer is really problematic. The media doesn't help, of course. All this "Kylie gets the all clear" stuff. In truth, I'm afraid, with this kind of cancer there simply is no all clear.'

'So it's five years until remission,' I repeated, crestfallen.

'Let me fetch you a box of tissues,' said Glamorous Assistant. I hadn't realised my tears were falling until she made the suggestion.

P and I said nothing while she nipped into the room next door. We didn't even look at each other; just tightened our grip while my mind wandered sarcastically to all the things that would happen before I could be moved from red to amber alert. There'd be a General Election. The London-hosted Olympic Games. Jamie's thirtieth. 'Christ,' I thought, 'Miley Cyrus will have done a stint in rehab, made a sex tape, squeezed out an illegitimate baby and written her memoirs by the time I'm in remission. This fucking thing goes on for ever.'

'Are you okay?' asked Glamorous Assistant, handing me a box of Kleenex.

'Not really, no.'

'It's just never ending,' added P, taking the words out of my mouth. 'We hoped there'd be some closure from today.'

'A lot of patients find this one of the hardest parts,' she said, which was simultaneously true and unhelpful, rather like being told, 'Well, you've got breast cancer. But so have loads of other people.'

'It's not hard,' I wept, now bawling uncontrollably. 'It's TORTUROUS. I can't sleep, I can't think straight, I can't get on with my life. And it's all I want to do.'

P slipped his arm around me. I suspected he was crying too, but I didn't look up to check.

'IT'S ALL I WANT TO DO!' I wailed again, suddenly realising how loud I had become. 'And it won't let me do it!'

'Believe me,' said Glamorous Assistant, pulling her chair closer towards us, 'there's nothing I'd like more than to tell you that everything is fine now, and to pack you off and say there's no need for you to come back. But it just doesn't work like that. And I wish for your sake that it did.' There was no doubting her compassion, and I wondered for a moment why she'd ever decided to go into a job like this. 'But I want to be able to help you in any way I can,' she continued. 'So perhaps I can help you with your sleeping, and then things might get easier?'

'What do you think, babe?' asked P.

'I don't know, I don't know,' I repeated, all in the same breath. 'I'm just continually paranoid that there's more cancer I don't know about. I have to know for sure that there's nothing else there. You need to tell me for certain that the treatment has worked.'

'I don't understand,' said a puzzled Glamorous Assistant.

'Can I have another CT scan?' I asked, fixing her with my eyes to demonstrate my seriousness.

'But why would you want another one?' she asked. 'Your pre-chemo scan was clear, was it not?'

'Yes, but what if something else has happened in the meantime?' I said, making less sense with every snivelled word. 'What if there's another tumour? What if there are more cells? I need to know. I can't relax until I know. It's imperative that I find out.'

I didn't like being reduced to this, and it wasn't pretty. I had assumed that a clear CT scan would be the little bit of finality I'd earned after the last few months. But, as it turned out, it wouldn't tell me a sodding thing.

'A CT scan can't pick up random cancer cells,' explained Glamorous Assistant. 'And it would be pointless to give you another CT scan now when your previous one was clear.'

'Can I pay for one?' I asked, though I wasn't entirely sure what with. 'Because if it comes back I want to know immediately so I can do something about it before it gets to this stage again.'

'Okay, let's talk this through,' she continued with calm in her voice which, I assumed, she wanted me to emulate. 'Even if a future CT scan were to pick up on a recurrence of this cancer, I'm afraid it wouldn't affect the outcome.'

This was the point at which P and I finally met eyes. Despite being seven arduous months into our encounter with The Bullshit, in that moment it hit us that we still knew a pitiful amount about how it worked. Because, as Glamorous Assistant explained, if there ever was a relapse of The Bullshit in my breast, there wouldn't be a damn thing they could do to cure it. They could manage it, and hopefully slow its progress – but never cure it.

With little regard for the other patients who were waiting to see her, we stayed with Glamorous Assistant for another half-hour or so, as she took us through the characteristics of grade-three cancer, what having had it would mean for me and what I'd need to do to manage the situation for the rest of my life. I'm sure it was exactly the same stuff that Smiley Surgeon had told us at a different hospital on the day we learned I had a tumour in my breast, but back then neither of us were in a position to take it in. Now, we were seeing the picture in full Technicolor, and having been through the treatment didn't make the reality any easier to stomach.

If only cancer were just a disease that you discover, get upset about, treat, then get over. Someone once told me that, upon her diagnosis, her consultant said, 'I don't want to frighten you, but you need to understand that your life will never be the same again.' And yet here we were, gunning for the finish-line, eager to get back to the lovely life we once knew. But we couldn't, because life had changed.

Up until that day, I had been careful of how I came across in front of the medical professionals who were charged with nursing me back to post-cancer fitness. But that Friday afternoon, I lost not just my patience, but also my ability to give a shit – so rather than the cheery, polite (or brown-nosing, in Smiley Surgeon's case) young woman that usually turned up to these appointments, Glamorous Assistant got her prickly, distraught, screw-up sister. And given that, I suppose it's no surprise that she chose to send me home with a prescription for antidepressants: another thing in my long list of Things I Said I'd Never Do.

I took the pill as soon as I got home from the hospital that evening, and then settled down with a cup of tea to write a cathartic blog post about the hospital visit that was already making me wince in shame at my angry, ranting, mentally unstable behaviour. But by the time I'd finished writing, I was seeing the world through a Chemical Brothers video, watching as my slippers doubled up, bouncing off the walls on my way to be sick and struggling to recognise my husband (who had to type up the remainder of the drafted blog post when I zonked out). What began as unpleasant quickly turned into something much scarier. If the drugs were supposed to calm my nerves and keep me from panicking, they were about as effective as a fart in a tornado.

The following morning, anxiously trying to hold myself together for my mate Jonze's wedding, I handed over the car keys to P who, strictly speaking, should have been on a drinking green card for the day. But even some twelve hours after taking the antidepressant, I was shaky, struggling to focus and generally a bit on the loopy side. Needless to say, the remainder of pills found their way into London's sewerage system. I had hated having to take one in the first place. But now I knew how they were capable of making me feel, I hated the thought of taking another one even more. But more than that – with a clearer head the following morning, I was as sure as I could be that I simply didn't need them.

Given that just eight months previous, I was having a lovely, carefree, Corona-filled time in Mexico, and I was now flat out in pyjamas on my sofa, recovering from some pretty hardcore cancer treatment, I think a few flip-outs can be forgiven. But after hearing about my new kind of prescription, people were suddenly over-concerned about me – not least my folks. ('How are *you* today? Really? But how are you in *yourself*?') Clearly, the word 'anti-depressant' set off the same alarms in their heads as it did in mine, and I could see them making all the wrong conclusions. 'Is she depressed? Should we go easy on her? Do you think we ought to say that?' When Mum and Dad visited us the following week, I made some God-awful low-fat cookies that were tantamount to eating chocolate-chip jiffy-bags, and yet nobody dared admit how bad they were. It infuriated me. What made me even tetchier were the presumptions about my mental state, and my crabbiness was giving people even more reason to think that I was depressed.

And so, with the knowledge that my family were more likely to believe what I wrote than what I said, I took to my blog. 'Let me say this for the record,' I announced. 'I. Am. Not. Depressed. What I *am* is shell-shocked and pissed off and actually pretty angry (still) that The Bullshit chose me from its one-in-three line-up. And, I'll admit, all of those crappy feelings have made me prone to the occasional mood swing. But I'm not suddenly teetering on the brink of despair. Of course there's nothing wrong with being depressed; there's no shame in it. I'm just not, is all. I'd be equally narked if you tried to tell me I preferred The Stones to The Beatles, that I was bad at spelling or that I was a Nottingham Forest fan. Now there's a thing to send a girl to the brink.'

CHAPTER 29

Restoration

February 2009

The last time we saw Smiley Surgeon it was snowing, and Central London looked as beautiful as I'd ever seen it. The usually busy waiting room at the hospital was deserted thanks to cancelled appointments, and the reception staff were giddy with the work-light excitement of two kids who'd been snowed out of school. P and I arrived early (only the second time in my life I've managed this; the first being our wedding day) and bagged the best seats directly outside the door to Smiley Surgeon's consultation room.

He's got a tough job, old SS. In one appointment he's telling someone they have breast cancer, the next he's congratulating them on getting so far through it (or, better still, letting them know there's nothing to worry about). And, from the looks on the faces of the couple who saw him immediately before us, that woman had clearly been thrown down the rabbit-hole of the former category.

She stared straight ahead as she walked out of the room on auto-pilot, subconsciously tearing the edges off a crumpled tissue. Her husband followed close behind, his hand resting helplessly in the small of her back, carrying his wife's coat and handbag because it was the only helpful thing he could do. And, just as we did after hearing the same news, they turned left out of SS's door and walked towards a room down the corridor where a core biopsy would be done to assess the extent of her tumour. As I wondered whether the woman would also come to loathe watercolour paintings as a result of the artwork on the wall of that room, I tutted, shook my head and turned to P. 'Poor sods,' I whispered. 'They won't be able to enjoy the snow now.'

But, for P and me at least, London looked even more beautiful when we came out of our appointment, having heard from Smiley Surgeon that he was impressed with my attitude throughout treatment (I didn't reveal the extent of my rant last week) and that my radiated skin was healing well enough for him to book in a date for my first reconstructive surgery. A vote of confidence from SS is like getting a gold star from the teacher you've been busting your gut to suck up to all term. And since it's no secret how much I adore the man, I'm not embarrassed to boast about it. (Ner ner ner ner ner.)

And so, the chapter-ending goal of Operation New Tit has been scheduled. I'll be going in for the main part in a month's time – that's the surgery to ensure a better shape for my boob (at the moment I fear it looks like a clenched fist), fit me with an A-list implant worthy of a modest-busted Dolly Parton ('fit' is the wrong terminology, I'm sure – that makes me sound like a BMW going in for a service), and create a new nipple. And that's the part that fascinates me most.

In short, what Smiley Surgeon will be doing is lifting the skin that lies where my nipple was (the skin that originally came from my back), then twisting it into a point which he'll fix in place to form a small mound that pretty much matches the height of my right nipple. It'll be higher than a bee sting, but flatter than a coconut macaroon. More of a nub, I suppose. (A nupple, if you will.) As Smiley Surgeon described this to me (not in confectionery terms, I should add), he opened his suit jacket slightly and mimed the process by pointing to his own nipple, in much the same way that you might say 'spiral staircase' and do that twirly motion with your index finger. I couldn't help but titter like a pubescent boy at the back of the class. P looked mortified.

Right now, here in my white vest, I look like the second image in a spot-the-difference game. Something's wrong with the picture, but you can't quite put your finger on what. But, like a once-glorious but now destroyed building, I'm slowly being restored to my former glory. A bit like The Hawley Arms after the Camden fire. It'll never be quite the same again, but hopefully the regulars won't be put off going back.

*

Thanks to my poorly timed panic attacks and our appointment with the Glamorous Assistant putting paid to any end-of-treatment revelry, P and I decided instead to celebrate something different: normality. With a month before my reconstructive surgery, we had a welcome break from hospital visits in which to stick a middle finger up to The Bullshit in the only way we knew how, and so we did our darndest to get on with normal life.

Having seen lots of our family over the past few months thanks to them being around to help out whenever necessary, it was time to get reacquainted with our friends, and so we invited a bunch of them round for a bit of an open-house at our flat one Saturday. It was an opportunity to catch up with all the people who'd been wanting to visit, but who we hadn't been able to see because The Bullshit got in the way. It was what my mum would call a 'gathering'. But then she'll do anything to avoid the word 'party'. Gathering implies Monopoly and Twiglets and the last tube home. Party implies gatecrashers and irritated neighbours and fag burns in the sofa. But, given our worktop-long row of spirit bottles, a table full of cava, the Beastie Boys played at volume and the fact that I was wearing heels indoors, I think we can safely label our get-together the latter. (We had Twiglets as well, mind. I mean, bloody hell, it's not a party without Twiglets. Not even a gathering.)

And, as is customary at parties, I got drunk. Which, I'm sure, is just a normal Saturday night to many of you. But not for this cancer patient. For me, getting drunk at home with mates was positively throw-your-TV-out-the-window, set-fire-to-a-million-quid, drive-a-car-into-a-swimming-pool rock 'n' roll. Of course having had The Bullshit hardly does wonders for your drinking prowess (making me the perfect credit-crunch date) and, judging by my mammoth hang-over the following day, it doesn't do an awful lot for your ability to shake it off, either. I felt sick, couldn't hold my brew for shaking, spoke in a voice that you could gravel a driveway with and had a head so painful I felt like I'd had a run-in with Mike Tyson. Man, I felt like hell. But it was the sweetest hangover I'd ever had.

Since June, whenever I'd felt like shit, it had been for an equally shitty reason. But feeling like shit because I'd drunk too much (translation: a modest amount for most people) was marvellous; my emancipatory rebirth into normal life. And, baby, I worked it. I went to bed in full make-up. I made a grease-tastic bacon, egg and tomato ketchup sandwich when I got up. I watched sport on the sofa in the clothes I fell asleep in, then retired to my mattress when sitting upright became too much effort. I watched the *Sex and the*

City movie twice (second time with director's commentary) and ate an entire box of Green & Black's chocolates. By myself. I caught up on *Coronation Street* over a curry with egg fried rice *and* chips, then polished off the prawn crackers during an episode of *Shameless*. It was a glorious, lardy Sunday, and I went to bed early with a contented smile on my face, nestling my cheeks into a pillow of eyeliner-smudge and prawn-cracker dust. 'This,' I thought, 'is what normal people do.'

My flirt with normality didn't stop at the weekend. Just when I thought the reckless abandon of my cancer shackles had reached its Twiglet-eating, dancing-in-the-living-room pinnacle, I pushed ordinary life to its limits and went back to work for a few hours for the first time in months. And, lawks, things had changed since I'd been holed up in my Bullshit bubble. Lots of lovely Soho shops had closed. There was a new security code on the front door. Different faces sat at different desks. I had a new log-in. Same old weak tea in chipped mugs, mind, but there was something quite poetic about that. But while I was busy figuring out what had altered in the office, others there were more intrigued as to what had altered about *me*.

'So, having cancer,' asked Kath over a bowl of miso soup when she took me out for lunch that day, 'do you think it's changed you?'

Without really thinking, I immediately answered 'yes', and launched into a monologue about my newly lowered tolerance for tears, particularly on reality TV shows: whinging on *Masterchef* because you ballsed up your halibut and all you've ever wanted from life is to 'spread joy' with your food; crying at *American Idol* auditions because you've 'been through hell and back' to get to the second round; sobbing in front of Sralan on *The Apprentice* because being 'successful in business' (whatever that means) is your life's ambition.

'I mean, come on,' I said. 'Find some sodding perspective!'

'Ha! I reckon you're just the same girl you ever were,' smiled Kath.

But while that was pretty surface-skimming and flippant in answer, the 'have I changed?' question was one I spent a lot of time thinking about. Of course you could argue that everything changes you in one way or another. A different job changes you. A new handbag changes you. Hell, a good shit changes you. But I'm talking about the more profound changes. Am I a better person as a result of having cancer? Do I have a new-found gratitude for each dawn? Have I uncovered a cosmic significance to all of this? No. I don't have a new appreciation for the scent of a rose or the taste of champagne or the beauty of a discarded newspaper tumbling along a windy Soho pavement. Cancer may have made me many things, but spiritually enlightened ain't one of them. *Zen and the Art of Cancer* this is not.

I had the same cancer debrief in my last (and possibly final) session with Mr Marbles. After confirming that he was 100 per cent with me on the I'm Not Depressed, It's My Cancer Treatment debate (take that, antidepressants), he asked me to list the good things that had come out of the previous few months.

'*Nothing* good has happened as a result of this,' I spat.

'I'd challenge that,' he replied, in that lovely, non-committal therapist-speak that basically translates as 'stop talking shite'. And, of course, he was right, damn him. (Maybe he should form a tag-team with Always-Right Breast Nurse and go on *Who Wants To Be A Millionaire?*)

I just didn't want to give anyone the false impression that

breast cancer could in some way be a good thing. Nor did I want to give it credit for the better things that had come out of my cancer experience. So instead me and Marbles settled on a compromise: of course I've changed as a result of having breast cancer, and a number of pleasant things have undoubtedly come along as a consequence – but, with or without The Bullshit (just as with or without the therapy), I'd have got there eventually. Cancer was just the catalyst, is all. It just got me there faster. And, like taking the Heathrow Express instead of the tube, it cost me a fair bit more, too.

Foolishly, I tried to talk over the has-anything-good-come-from-cancer question with Jamie, too.

'Frankly, sis, I think you've done us all a favour,' he said on the phone the night before our treatment-is-over family trip to Rome. 'Because if you hadn't got cancer, we might not have been going away this weekend.'

'Riiight. So you're saying that my getting cancer was merely a selfless act to ensure that you got a mini-break?'

'Exactly. You orchestrated the whole thing. And, on behalf of the family, I'd like to say that we're very grateful.'

CHAPTER 30

What's my age again?

March 2009

Probably conscious that its days are numbered, I've been taking the wig option more often of late, despite the fact that what's growing underneath makes wearing it even more uncomfortable. Plus, I reckon I'll miss making that relieved 'ahh' noise whenever I take it off. (Also applicable to being released from handcuffs, the first sip of lager on a hot day and taking off your high heels in the cab home.) Back in my early wig-wearing days – when my hair was falling out fast, but I wasn't quite bald (the Bobby Charlton stage, if you will) – I bought a little lycra cap that's specially designed for wig-wearers to flatten what remains beneath the syrup, ensuring a better wig-fit. It was a bit like pulling a pop sock over my head. If I'd yanked it down over my eyes, I'd have been one swag bag and a stripy jumper away from turning into a cartoon bank robber. But the pop sock worked, and I suspect that, if I keep up the current wig-wearing status quo with the barnet I'm now growing, I'll be forced to head back to one of the wig shops I swore I'd never again set foot in to buy myself a new hair-flattening device.

I've not ditched the headscarf altogether. It's just that, lately, I've found myself in a few wig-necessary situations. Passport control, for one. What's the protocol on hair loss and passport photos? (See, *that's* the kind of thing those 'welcome to cancer' leaflets should tell you. I want practicalities, dammit, not a namby-pamby side-panel on 'understanding your emotions'.) In my passport photo, I'm a tanned lass with long, blonde hair (who, inexplicably, looks like she's overdone the valium). But the reality now is, of course, different (I look like I've overdone the Veet). So does that necessitate a new passport photo? Would they stop me if I went through airport security in a headscarf, and publicly humiliate me by forcing me to run it through the X-ray machine with my boots, then carry it on board in a see-through plastic bag? Are headscarves now up there with matches, tweezers and copies of the Qur'an as terrorist-suspicion-arousing signals?

All of this only occurred to me the night before our trip to Rome so, to save my blushes, I reached for the rug in the hope that it'd just look like I'd had a haircut, and not had my head shaved by some loony School For Terrorists. Not that the wig stopped me acting suspiciously when I handed over my passport, mind. I put on my very best show of I-get-on-flights-to-Italy-all-the-time nonchalance (chewing gum + headphones + fiddling with iPhone = seasoned traveller), but couldn't do much to disguise the shaking hands, sweaty palms and hot flush. They let me through anyway, of course. I'm sure even airport security staff would rather mess with a terrorist than an early-menopausal woman.

Then there's the recommended wig-wearing business of being a tourist in Rome. And not just because I suspect the fashion-conscious Italians would be more receptive to a Hermès headscarf than my H&M one. Nope, tourism = photo-taking, and I was buggered if I was going to look back on family photos of everyone gathered around an obvious-looking cancer patient posing unsteadily outside the Colosseum, like a doddery old dear on day release from the nursing home. There are very few photos in existence of me in a headscarf, and I'm keeping it that way.

All that said, I found out the hard way that certain city-sightseeing situations are less rug-receptive than others. Tourism Tip For Cancer Patients #1: wigs and open-top buses don't mix.

*

'Did you tell your family you were going to do this?' asked Tills.

'And ruin a lovely weekend in Rome? God no.'

'But your mum's going to freak, no?'

'Probably, yeah. But bugger it, Tills. I'm doing this for me. Anyway, it's pretty daft that I'm nearly thirty and sitting here worrying about what my mum's going to think.'

'Yeah, maybe. But it's also pretty daft that you're having hot flushes at thirty, too,' she said, handing me a magazine to fan myself with as we drank our coffee.

'So I'm doing it,' I said.

'You're really doing it,' repeated Tills.

Being able to get back to the kind of chatting-over-coffee, weekend-away familiarity that I'd been craving for so long was undoubtedly wonderful, but in many ways it also served as a reminder of just how much had altered before I had been able to get that normality back. When your life has changed in such a gargantuan way, there's a sense of wanting to change something else to reflect it – be it your haircut or your career or your relationship. And so, with my hair still stalling, my job ready and waiting for me to return to and my marriage on the Not-To-Be-Messed-With list, I guess that's how I ended up leaving that coffee shop with Tills and walking into a tattoo studio.

Since treatment finished, I had been thinking a lot about my mum's favourite poem – 'Warning', by Jenny Joseph – and its subject of growing old in outrageous style. Thanks to a sudden inability to know how to act my age, I especially identified with the line 'and make up for the sobriety of my youth'. Here was I planning debauched weeks at Glastonbury and rapping into my toothbrush one moment; then the next turning purple from a hot flush as my mate fanned me with a copy of *Take a Break*. It was time to do something about it.

And yes, getting a tattoo was probably fifteen years too late for teenage rebellion. But then, I figured, nothing about my ageing process was working to rule any more, so going from a hot flush to an ink-filled needle seemed strangely appropriate. That morning, an hour's menopause-related Googling had confirmed that it was the right thing to do. During my search, I discovered a 'menopause scoresheet', on which you could log the severity of your symptoms and learn . . . well, nothing you didn't already know. But at the top of the page was an image of three smiling fifty-something women, by way of we're-all-in-it-together reassurance. One of them was even wearing sports gear, clearly in preparation for an afternoon of tea and tennis at the Menopausal Ladies' Club, of which I was now a scoresheet-approved member.

The trouble was, despite the infuriating hot flushes, the difficulty sleeping, the change in my skin, the loss of my periods and the joint aches of a woman twice my age, I considered myself more *Mean Girls* than *Calendar Girls*, and in no way was I ready for my Menopausal Ladies' Club welcome pack.

Just like breast cancer and wig-wearing, I had always assumed menopause to be one of those things that I'd have to worry about many years down the line. So now, with the mind of a twenty-nine-year-old but the body of a fifty-nine-year-old, for the first time in my life, I struggled to know how to behave. In many ways, getting a tattoo punctuated the end of my old Grand Life Plan and the beginning of a new – infinitely less rigid – one. Or perhaps that's all the therapy talking, and it is what it is – a star-shaped bit of ink.

I still like to think, though, that my star marks the full stop to many a sentence: the end of my active treatment (it's on my right wrist, beside the point at which my chemo needles were inserted), the reward for getting through those difficult few months (it's no coincidence that the shape isn't unlike that of the star stickers that primary teachers award their pupils), plus the recognition that my life has changed irreparably, and that Solomon Grundy life plans aren't all they're cracked up to be.

Still, I'm pleased that I stuck to the old plan for as long as I was able. I'm glad I was a Good Girl. It got things done. But now there was no plan to speak of – just a new tattoo and a blank page. And, while that terrified and excited me in equal measure, I was intrigued to see what would come next, once Operation New Tit was done with.

The life-planners were out in force on the day Tills and I went to get my tattoo, as we discovered over a celebratory post-ink drink in a department-store restaurant. There we were, strutting in with our designer handbags while other women our age struggled in with designer prams. We clinked beer bottles while they shook milk bottles. We talked tattoos while they talked toddlers. And while, several months previous, I'd have been envious of the women on the tables surrounding us, I realised there was a lot to like about my screwed-up approach to age. Benjamin Button eat your heart out – this was The Curious Case of Lisa Lynch. And so, in honour of my fucked-up, twenty-something menopause, I wrote my own 'Warning'.

When I am thirty I shall have a short, punky haircut
And wear high-street frocks with Louboutin heels.
I shall spank my Premium Bonds on pedicures and
   shiny Mac gadgets
And five-star holidays, and flip the bird to my pension.
I shall teach my friends' kids filthy jokes
And swear at traffic wardens and wink at builders
And flirt with shy-looking teenage waiters
And pretend I'm in an episode of *Skins*.
I shall show off my tattoo in cropped-sleeve jackets
And wear glittery make-up to the supermarket
And learn to rap.

CHAPTER 31

Dotting the i

Is there a Guinness World Record entry for the world's biggest nipple? Because I think I've got it. For verification purposes, I suppose it's strictly a nupple. And since there aren't even half as many nupples in the world as there are nipples, I'm skipping the adjudication and taking the crown. Well done me.

I've only caught a very quick glimpse of it, mid morphine-trip from my hospital bed when a nurse came to inspect my wounds (it might have been the drugs, but I'm sure her name badge said 'Mariwana'), but even in my stoned state I couldn't believe what I'd seen beneath the bloody dressings. Sheesh, it could have taken my eye out. Seriously, it's the size of a grape. It's not just the small mound I'd expected from Phase One of Operation New Tit, but in fact a fully-fledged, proud-as-punch, specially constructed imitation erect nipple. I know! Erect! Hell, that's not even something I can say for my right nipple. That's generally a lazy little bugger, only standing to attention when absolutely necessary. Not so the nupple. This little baby (sorry, big baby) belongs on a newsagent's top shelf. Or, better still, beneath a smutty bikini in a *Carry On* film. (Oh behave.)

Actually, I fear it might be better suited to a horror film right now, given the stitching and swelling and scabbing. Always-Right Breast Nurse came to visit me on the ward before my surgery to explain the procedure, forewarning me that the new nip would be 'a bit on the large side' post-surgery, as Smiley Surgeon purposely intended to make it bigger than it would actually end up. Since it's not made from living tissue, part of it will eventually die and fall off like the leftover bit of umbilical cord on a baby's belly button.

It was a brilliant surprise, seeing Always-Right Breast Nurse. Given that she doesn't usually work on Saturdays, I hadn't expected to see her on the day of my surgery, and her visit to my hospital bed was the one calming tactic that actually worked on me. In many ways, heading back into hospital felt like the same old cancer-treatment routine: turning my nervous frustration into shouting at P the night before (this time about getting the blinds to sit straight, or some other such nonsense), blocking the loo before leaving home, sobbing on the cab journey there, then blocking the loo again when I got to the hospital (what can I say – nerves do funny things to your bowels). It was a surreal, emotional experience, being led back to the same ward where I'd spent several days last June, for the removal of what was about to be replaced. Both Smiley Surgeon and Always-Right Breast Nurse mentioned that the months seemed to have passed so quickly since the last time we were discussing my left breast on a hospital ward. And I suppose it does seem speedy to them. They're doing this kind of thing every day, but for me it's been a lengthy, loathsome, laborious process that's gifted me my first grey hairs. ('No bloody wonder,' said Dad as he pulled them from my head.)

No amount of pre-op nerves could make me behave around Smiley Surgeon when he came to visit me before his Saturday-afternoon melon-twisting session, mind. I was my usual, cringe-worthy, goony self. Actually, I was worse than that. I was a complete twat. He poked his head around the door and – this being the first time he'd seen me without long hair, a wig or a headscarf – for a second he didn't recognise me. 'Wow, your hair!' he exclaimed, realising that he was in the right place and walking towards me purposefully with his clipboard.

'Huh, yeah,' I snorted embarrassingly. (Goon alert . . .) 'Hey, look!' I yawped, pointing at his head. 'I'm catching you up!' From the corner of my eye, I saw P wince as his head fell into his hands, and felt my face getting hotter as I kicked myself for being more of a tit than the body part that Smiley Surgeon was about to create.

Normally I'm a think-before-you-speak kind of girl, but whenever I'm around this man, I just cannot stop these ridiculous things from spewing out of my mouth. It's like trying to act cool around a Beatle. Though I'm sure I'd be more composed around Paul McCartney than I am around Smiley Surgeon. Hell, compared to how I am with him I reckon I'd be a picture of ease if I ever met the Queen or the Dalai Lama or Dave Grohl. Well, maybe not Grohl. The man is a legend. Whereas I, on the other hand, am a twonk.

As he always does so expertly, Smiley Surgeon delicately side-stepped my fame-blinded faux pas (surely the breast reconstruction equivalent of 'I carried a *watermelon*?'), quickly moving on to the business of Operation New Tit. He stood opposite me as I sat topless on my hospital bed, sizing up my real boob against my meantime-boob, and explaining that he didn't think size and weight would be a problem, but that he might have to spend some time getting the projection right (which, I think, was a polite way of saying that my boobs are a good shape, but they don't stick out all that much). Apparently, in preparation for the surgery, he lines up all the available implants in the relevant cup size, then tries out the likeliest ones after he's made the incision before settling on the one that'll stay beneath my skin. I loved the thought of Smiley Surgeon standing behind a table filled with size-ordered fake tits, like a bell-ringer ready to perform, and I focused on that image as the anaesthetist sent me off to sleep.

When I woke up three hours later, I caught myself mumbling P's name (thank God it wasn't Smiley Surgeon's) as the anaesthetist who'd put me under handed me a tissue to wipe my tears. I was utterly overwhelmed. There I lay, gowned up and drowsy from the drugs, in the same recovery room I awoke in after my mastectomy, directly opposite the same silver clock and surrounded by the same familiar smells of detergent and dressings that I hadn't realised I'd remembered from last time.

I cried quietly all the way back to the ward, too, and even once I was back in my bed. I couldn't help it. It wasn't necessarily out of pain or discomfort; more out of anguish. Trauma, even. I was shell-shocked by the months of treatment I'd been through to get to this point, yet completely surprised that I'd finally – *finally* – made it here. The whole experience was unexpectedly turning into a bitter reminder of everything I'd fought so hard to forget, and the disbelieving, impossible-to-stomach impact of my diagnosis was hitting me all over again.

Thankfully, P knew just the trick to put a stop to my tears and, perching on the side of my bed, produced a tiny Tiffany bag that brought me round from my morphine-induced sobbing-stupor faster than you can say 'bling'. Inside the little bag was a card that read: *For my wonderful wife, a wonderful ring to mark our wonderful future.* Of course that set me off all over again, even before I'd seen what was in the box.

'Well,' said P, gesturing to my new tit, 'you've gone through all this to give me something new to play with. The least I can do is give you the same in return.' And what a deal! I'm going to snag some tights on this baby, I tell you. He's right; it *is* wonderful. A sparkling, proud-standing and fabulously show-

245

offy cocktail ring to wear on my middle finger – our way of sticking one up to The Bullshit. I can't help but think that P's got the raw end of the deal, though. After all, his toy's going to shrink. But not mine. Mine's staying middle-finger-erect for ever.

*

The week before my surgery it was Lil's thirtieth, and I used her party to mark my last night of wig-wearing. And, just like the first time I wore it, it was all a bit of an anticlimax. I had visions of strutting out of the pub and getting a mate to animatedly tear it off my head in the middle of Soho, freaking out the drag queens to the sound of trumpets and adoring applause from the revellers of W1 (seems I'm more drama queen than drag queen). In fact, it wasn't quite as liberating as I'd have hoped. I was narked and sweaty from a hot-flush-filled evening, and struggling to hold myself upright in my sky-high peep-toes, so out of practice was I at the business of Central London socialising. So the rug was not ripped off to an emancipatory, horn-section sound-track; it was instead done by P to an exasperated, car-horn chorus as I attempted to three-point-turn my way out of a tricky parking space. Which pretty much summed up my entire experience as a wig-wearer: clumsy, begrudging and not a little embarrassing.

The original plan had been to stick with headscarves (or the wig, on special occasions) for another couple of months. But even I knew that it would be too much of a hassle to keep up the pretence in hospital and so I figured this was as good a time as any to out myself as a very-short-haired person. Upon asking my family and friends what to do with my baldness-covering devices, the overwhelming consensus was to throw them away in spectacular fashion. Firing them from a cannon or sending them off on a burning log out to sea or some such. Both of which sounded very appealing, were it not for the fact that I was completely terrified that the moment I decided to ditch them, I'd discover that they were still needed. And so, even as I write this, with a decent head of hair and several months after having relegated Wig 1 to a bottom drawer, that's exactly where it remains – in my bottom drawer, tangled up in the unruly chaos of hairbrushes and headbands. It's ruined, of course. But for some reason I can't bring myself to throw it away.

With my bag packed and my ill-person pyjamas washed and ironed by Mum (still keeping to her promise of helping to ease these moments in the best way she knew how), everything was ready for Operation New Tit. Well, everything except me. This was the part I'd been waiting for – the chance finally to get back the beautiful breast that cancer had taken from me. And while I understood the surgery was nothing like as serious as my previous operation, that the reason for this procedure was a more welcome one, and that the hospital stay wouldn't be as long, I had still switched from kid-on-Christmas Eve excited to night-before-exam-results brick-shitting.

I knew that my nervousness was bordering on the irrational, and I knew the reason why. The last time I came around from my anaesthetic, Smiley Surgeon came to my bed with the news that my cancer had spread. And I couldn't help but prepare myself for bad news when I woke up this time, too. I hated not knowing what was going on in my body. It's not that I knew exactly what was happening in there pre-Bullshit either, of course, but now it was driving me to obsession.

Everyone was quick to tell me that it would be okay, that

there was nothing to worry about, that I should just focus on the end result. But, as well as trying to avoid the surgery-subject by snapping at people instead, I was actively trying *not* to think about the end result. I didn't want to get my hopes up, like I did about the wig-buying. Back then, I wanted the perfect replica of my original hair. And now, I wanted the perfect replica of my original boob. But I'd learned my lesson; I knew I wasn't going to get it. The wig may have been poker-straight and frizz-free and kink-proof, but it wasn't *my* hair. And I was worried that I'd feel the same way about the specially constructed, all-singing, all-dancing Super Tit that Smiley Surgeon was going to spend his Saturday afternoon crafting. (Remember when Carrie Bradshaw lost her treasured 'Carrie' nameplate necklace and the little Russian dude bought her a diamond one to replace it? Now substitute the 'Carrie' necklace with my old tit, and the diamond necklace with my new tit, and you've got the idea. Note to self: *Sex and the City* = not real life.)

Before my surgery, though, was an operation for Sgt Pepper, when we took her to be spayed. And even that was traumatic. It was a window into what it must have been like for P and Jamie and my parents during my eight-hour mastectomy. I was a right bloody mess while she was at the vet's – waiting nervously by the phone, trying to keep busy by writing a blog post (which I later binned, utter shit that it was), spilling my tea down the side of the sofa, chewing off what was left of my fingernails.

So, as I concluded last time, in many ways I was going to have the easy part: I'd be knocked out, none the wiser while my family counted the minutes, drank endless cups of tea and tried to busy themselves. Fortunately, unlike Sgt Pepper, I wouldn't be coming round from my operation to find a plastic cone around my neck. Though, when I woke up after the op, I was relieved to discover something rather cone-shaped beneath the left side of my hospital gown.

Earlier that morning, I had taken a sneaky photo of my Old Tit on my iPhone. And even through my hospital gown I could see that the 'after' photo was going to be a hell of a lot more impressive.

'So, what do you think of it?' beamed a proud Smiley Surgeon, staring intently at my chest as I walked into his room for my post-op check-up a week later. (I had become so used to folk staring at my tits that I was becoming quite offended when people out in the Real World spoke to my face.) Carefully avoiding my usual levels of goondom but inexplicably turning scouse in the process, I replied in an oddly high-pitched voice. 'I'm made up, la!' (Okay, so I just added the 'la' for dramatic effect, but still. What was my problem?)

'Oh-kaay. Let's have a look,' he replied, side-stepping my comedy accent and gesturing to the bed behind the curtain.

Always-Right Breast Nurse was on hand to remove my dressings and, for the first time since the sneaky look in my hospital bed, I got to see the full glory of my newly formed nupple. Not to mention the beautiful, perfectly round mound that it sat atop, like an especially delicious cherry bakewell or iced bun. While SS prodded at my new boob and I looked on admiringly (at him *and* the New Tit), I couldn't help but think of the *Generation Game*. Believe me, if Brucie had handed you a lump of clay and a pottery wheel and given you sixty seconds to create a breast, Smiley Surgeon would have been the visiting expert whose model you had to copy. (Didn't he do well?)

Undoubtedly the sweetest part of my check-up, however, was watching SS's smiling face (P is convinced he only smiles for me, by the way, and that he's more Serious Surgeon with his other patients) as he explained that, mid-surgery, he'd had a 'good look around in there'. (That, rather flatteringly, makes my tit sound like Mary Poppins' handbag, when I'm sure that a 'good look around' my B-cup is actually tantamount to a twenty-second shufty.) But he continued with a sentence that ended in those few little words that every girl dreams of hearing: '. . . no sign of cancer.' I'd been too afraid to ask him what he'd discovered while inside my boob, for fear of letting slip my vision of an Alien-style tumour bursting out and creating havoc in the operating theatre, so I was as pleased that he'd picked up on my unspoken worry as I was about the words he'd said. No. Sign. Of. Cancer. Forget 'cellar door' – *these* are the most beautiful words in the English language.

But, beautiful as those words were, hearing them was strangely unsettling. I didn't know what to say, plumping for a simple, 'Phew,' and heading out of my appointment in an uncharacteristically timid manner. You'd think that hearing the words 'no sign of cancer' would have you doing backflips across the kitchen. And beside the fact that (a) it would hurt too much, (b) I can't do a backflip, and (c) even if I could, the size of our kitchen would mean me crashing into a wall mid-air, that's oddly not how you feel you ought to react. It's weirdly anticlimactic, which is a lesson you'd think I'd have learned, given the many stalling, false finishes I'd come to expect of The Bullshit.

So, despite his words, I worked myself up into a panic after recounting to my family and friends the words that Smiley Surgeon had told me. Was I speaking too soon? Should I shut up about it? I thought I was healthy once before – was The Bullshit going to come back to bite me on the ass again? I hated raining on my own parade in this way, because, hell, this was amazing news. Better than that – it was the best news in the history of the known world. But it was also just another false finish.

It's a question of semantics – something in which the medical world is deviously skilled, and in which I was hurriedly having to coach other people.

'Wow! You're cancer free!' they'd say.

'Um, not exactly, no,' I'd say.

'But your surgeon said . . .?'

'He said there was no sign of cancer in my left breast.'

'And isn't that the same thing?'

'Unfortunately not, no.'

Bloody cancer. It's a whole other language. And just as everyone around me figured they'd got the gist of it, in I'd swoop with my medical clarifications to hand them a D grade and put right their mistakes, like an annoying pedant who corrects everyone's grammatical errors. (Oh, hang on, I'm that too.) I had no choice but to put them right, though. Because 'no sign of cancer' does not mean 'cancer free'. Once you've had cancer, there is no 'cancer free'.

But at the time, simply liking and lumping it fell disappointingly short of the mark. I wanted to scream, 'I did it!' I wanted to tell people that I 'beat' breast cancer. I wanted to refer to it in the past tense. But bloody, sodding, know-all medical science dictates that I can *never* say that. As I've said a hundred times before, there is no definite cure for breast cancer. There is no 'all clear'. And so you've got to be happy with second place on the podium. (Kind of how I felt after Derby lost to Leicester in the play-off final of 1994, and I've still not got over that.)

That didn't mean that there was nothing to celebrate, of course. The 'it' in 'I did it' just meant something different, is all. It meant that I'd seen off six successful sessions of chemo, twenty-eight successful sessions of radio, the first stage of a successful reconstruction, and that I was successfully edging ever closer to leading a more normal life. And since we all know from bitter experience that not everyone gets to celebrate those kind of successes, I decided that I was going to enjoy the moment as best I could. And so, from a lack of rooftops to scream from, I took to my blog and shouted it there instead: 'I did it! I fucking did it!'

CHAPTER 32

Fitting image

April 2009

The last time I used my hair straighteners, I sat on them. Not with a quick glance of a jeans pocket, but flat onto bare skin, arse cheeks expertly manoeuvring themselves over the 100-degree aluminium, then lowering down carefully like a fairground grab-a-prize game. I dare say it was nature's way of calling my hair-straightening proceedings to a halt. Because, in my quest to make good the hair that remained on my head, I wasn't so much sleekening my locks as giving alopecia a helping hand.

Adding insult to balding injury was the corker of a burn it left on my right bum-cheek; a branding from the tribe of GHD. Two angry, parallel lines, each about three inches long, ensuring that the least attractive part of my body was granted another blemish to compete with my cellulite for unwanted beachside attention. I showed P and my folks the damage when my squeals beckoned them in. 'You know what?' said Mum, ever keen to find the bright side. 'I'm sure it'll have gone by the time you need to use those straighteners again.' But, looking in the mirror when I got out of the shower last night, my short hair isn't the only reminder of my Bobby Charlton period. My steroid-sculpted behind also tells a tale. Because, half-hidden by my knicker line but nevertheless visible, the bum-brand remains. Not quite as angry as before, but still obvious enough to demonstrate my idiocy to whoever's on the next sunlounger.

Getting the straighteners out again turned out to be a tad premature, actually. It was a bit like the time I assured P I could rectify his short frizz after a ten-minute session with the appliance, but just ended up scalding his scalp. It's not that I'm not happy to embrace my new curls (hell, any hair is better than no hair), but right now my 'do is more Brillo pad than brill. And so this week I'll be spending the GDP of a small country on my first post-chemo cut and colour.

The advice is to wait six months after the date of your final chemo before putting any colour onto your hair. And although my appointment falls a fortnight short of that time, I'm hoping it won't matter, since I've carefully chosen an environmentally aware (and therefore rinse-your-wallet-dry expensive) salon with 97 per cent natural hair colourants. Plus, since it's been just shy of a year since I had a haircut I was happy with, I'm taking impatience to night-before-birthday levels and just. can't. wait. any. longer. In hideous hair terms, two weeks feels like several millennia.

You'd think that I'd have got used to my short crop by now, but it still surprises me when I catch sight of my reflection. In my mind's eye, I've still got hair like Jessica Rabbit. Not that I'd have admitted to that little boast before. Actually, 'admitted to' isn't right – I'd never have believed it. But it's funny how six sessions of chemo can change your mind. Now, when I look back at photos of Old Me, I realise that the ex-colleague I met in the pub not long before my diagnosis was right. Despite being perhaps the unlikeliest source of a compliment I'd ever known, he stood back and looked admiringly at my newly grown-out fringe. 'Bloody hell, lass,' he said, 'Your hair's looking gorgeous.' And he wasn't wrong.

My post-chemo hairdo comes as part of a carefully choreographed New Image Week, in which I'll also be seeing a Topshop style advisor (I haven't got a spring/summer stitch to wear, having thrown away much of last year's wardrobe in that tearful, post-diagnosis rage), as well as investing in red lipstick for the first time, enrolling at the Alice Cooper School of Eye-liner and disguising my pasty pallor with enough St Tropez to make me look like the spawn of an Oompa Loompa. And then there's some serious underwear shopping to be done, too. It's going to be an expensive week. (Is it okay to use the L'Oreal excuse with your bank manager? 'And why do you need this overdraft extension, Mrs Lynch?' 'Because I'm worth it.')

I'd love to tell you that all of this is about making myself feel better. Something I'm doing just for me, because I'm long overdue some self-attention, because I've earned it and because it's a damn good opportunity to test out all the looks I would never have been game enough to try pre-Bullshit. And while all of those things are indeed true, they're not the only reasons behind the New Me. (Truth is, breast cancer or no breast cancer, I can a-l-w-a-y-s find an excuse to shop.) Just like my tattoo, New Image Week is my way of sending a message to all of the many people I'll be seeing again in pubs and bars and cafés and restaurants and dining rooms and the office. It's a statement: 'Hello, I've changed.' Because there's no getting away from it. I *have* changed.

Not that the Old Me is completely dead and buried, mind. There might be a permanent star-shaped symbol of the New Me on the inside of my right wrist, but there'll always be a reminder of the girl I once was on my right buttock.

*

Much to my surprise, after ditching my headscarf, I wasn't automatically sporting the kind of coiffured crop that Kylie carried off so expertly. Instead, I had the barnet of a six-month-old baby. My hair looked like something that had happened to me. And I wanted my hair to look like *I'd* happened to *it*. So, with the help of a newsagent's worth of women's magazines, I decided to go blonde. Not blonde like before. Stand-up-and-take-notice blonde. Think Marilyn Monroe, Agyness Deyn, Gwen Stefani, or Gary Barlow circa 1992. That way, I figured, it would look like a hairdo that was done out of choice; on purpose – and not because cancer had forced its hairdressing hand. But by, heck, did I get it wrong.

It's funny what people say compared to what they mean. Whether it's 'we must catch up soon' or 'no, darling, your bum looks positively tiny', common courtesy dictates that it's better to avoid offending someone than it is to tell the truth. And it's a bloody good job. Because, after what I had assumed was an expertly planned image change, there was one question I just wasn't interested in the truthful answer to: 'How's my hair?'

'I love it,' said Tills. 'It's sexy.'

'I think I've made a terrible mistake,' I said as we drove from the hair appointment to my session with a Topshop style advisor.

'Nah, no way,' she said unconvincingly. 'It's just a massive change, that's all. But that's what you wanted, right?'

'I thought I did,' I replied, checking my bleached crop in the rear-view mirror. 'But now I've got it, I don't think I can carry it off.'

We'd spent a lovely girly morning at the salon, me and Tills. I'd treated her to a manicure by way of thanks for her unending support, we'd had a lovely lunch flicking through the weeklies for some fantasy clothes shopping, and we'd nattered all the way through my appointment, boring the arse off my colourist with daft stories about our cats. With Tills managing proceedings like some kind of bleaching invigilator, the colourist was careful to listen to everything I'd asked for and duly obliged. Things were going well. New Image Day was looking like a success, and with everyone around me being especially lovely and complimentary about the shock of short, platinum hair that was confidently contrasting with my black gown, there was no reason to feel anything other than chuffed. Finally, I had hair I'd *chosen* to have.

But, as the harsh light of day and several suspicious sideways glances expertly demonstrated, the hair I'd chosen didn't suit me. I might have wanted a funky, punky, peroxide, statement 'do, but Lady Gaga I ain't. And so my poker face lasted the distance from the hairdresser's to the Topshop changing room, where Tills took a few photos of my new crop on her mobile phone, and I collapsed into sobs when I saw them, just as I had when looking at the photo of a fat lass in a wig that Ant had posted on Facebook.

The fault was entirely my own. I had got what I'd asked for: the trendy, relevant, never-would-have-tried-it-otherwise look that would tell the world how I'd changed; how I was on top of cancer; how I was ready to take on anything that life threw at me. But what I'd asked for wasn't right. It wasn't hair that I'd *chosen* to have – if I could have chosen hair, I'd have had it exactly the way it was pre-Bullshit, and not have cancer force me into a pixie crop. And I had to confront the fact that actually, I just wasn't feeling feisty enough to carry off the look I'd thought I wanted. It was hair that stood out from the crowd – and, as it turned out, I didn't want to stand out. It was hair that screamed confidence – and I didn't have as much as I'd thought. It was hair that suggested its owner was cool, attractive, hot and edgy – and I'd never felt further from those things. I could talk the talk all I wanted, confidently proclaiming my new image to be the triumphant, cancer-beating look that was all mine, making me way cooler than the girl I was pre-Bullshit. But, having surrendered all the goods to back it up along with the hair I lost in the first place, this was categorically not the time to be cashing in on my confidence. It was the time to start slowly building it back up again.

Sobbing in a post-salon coffee stop with Tills and P either side of me, I kicked myself for learning nothing since the last time the three of us attempted to make the best of my hair-loss situation. 'Here we are again,' I thought, 'back at my first wig-buying experience.' Back then, I walked into the room expecting to skip out with something I loved as much as my original hair. And this time around, I'd expected exactly the same. Better yet, I wanted people to pass me in the street and think nothing of me. Not 'ooh, is she wearing a wig?' or 'crikey, she's young to be wearing a headscarf'. Not even 'wow, look how confidently she's carrying that crop'. Nothing. Because them thinking nothing would mean that I was no different to anyone else. And when it came down to it, *that* was the kind of normal I was after.

My problem wasn't just in failing to realise that a freckly gal needs something a bit warmer than bright, white hair. It was in allowing my expectations to run away with me. In my mind, I was going to walk out of that salon the new Agyness Deyn. Better than that, actually – I was going to walk out of there the New Me. I had built up New Image Day to be a defining moment in my escape from cancer's grip: the day on which I stopped being the girl with breast cancer, and started being the girl with the funky hair. The day on which I could stop hiding away, and return to the world with a bright, blonde bang. I'd even given it a name, for fuck's sake. New Image Day was going to be as significant a turning point as the day of my diagnosis or my mastectomy or my final chemo.

Almost eleven months into my experience of The Bullshit, and I still couldn't get my head around the fact that I wasn't in control. Cancer was in control. And no amount of new clothes or hair colourant or New Image Days could change that. The reality is that the milestones aren't the scripted occasions, but the seemingly insignificant rites of passage that you don't notice until they've passed. Washing your hair for the first time after losing it. Walking the length of your street without having to stop for a rest. Falling asleep without the help of sleeping pills. Catching yourself saying 'I've *had* cancer' instead of 'I've *got* cancer'. *These* are the things that matter. These are the things that make a difference. They're the niggling, nil-nil away draws that guarantee your safety at the end of the season. They're not pretty, they're not memorable, and they're definitely not going to make it onto *Match of the Day*, but they're vital nonetheless. They're the things I should have been blogging about, when instead I was more interested in the showy wonder-goals that would make for a better highlights package.

'When am I going to learn my lesson?' I asked Tills after we'd ditched my Topshop stylist for an emergency appointment with my second colourist of the day.

'You weren't to know how you'd feel, darling,' she reassured me. 'Besides, you wanted peroxide hair today, and you tried it. Now you can try something else too.'

259

The junior colourist looked at me as though I were a lunatic. 'Hang on – you only had this colour done today?'

'That's right,' snapped Tills, back in no-bullshit management mode. 'And she'd like it to be a bit less harsh, and a bit more warm. Are you able to do that?'

'Um, yeah. I s'pose so,' she conceded, heading across the salon to mix some more colour.

'Nobody talks about this part,' I complained to Tills over a mug of tea. 'People warn you how hard it is to get a diagnosis and go through chemo and lose your hair. But nobody ever warned me how hard it would be to get over treatment, or how long it takes to feel right after chemo, or how difficult it is to get your hair back. There isn't a leaflet for this stuff.'

But, then, how could there be? Hell, even now I wouldn't know how to tell someone who'd just been diagnosed that there's so much more tricky stuff to negotiate once treatment has finished; that you're suddenly left to deal with the gravity of what's happened to you; that you've somehow got to alter all of your expectations.

But harder than even doing those things is accepting that you've got to do them in the first place. Cancer changed my life, but I didn't want to have to change the way I lived to accommodate it. I didn't *want* to lower my expectations. I wanted to get excited and look forward and face my future with optimism. I wanted to plan ahead. I wanted to feel normal. I wanted to stop seeing cancer when I looked in the mirror. I wanted to take the credit for my crop. I wanted to turn the things that cancer was making me do into significant, fun moments that I was in control of. I wanted to turn The Bullshit into something brilliant.

The following morning – at my third hair appointment in the space of twenty-four hours – I poured out my heart to yet another hair colourist, who couldn't believe that I'd wanted such a drastic change of colour in the first place. 'You've always had long hair before this, yes?' he asked in his devastatingly sexy French accent.

'Mm-hmm,' I nodded.

'Then suddenly having short hair is enough of a new image for you! You don't need crazy blonde too,' he advised, before turning my hair just a couple of shades lighter than its natural colour.

And so there was no New Me.

But nor was there an Old Me.

There was just Me. Albeit with a little less hair (and a little more tit).

CHAPTER 33

A change of season

May 2009

I've always wished I had the kind of local that you could walk into, know everyone at the bar and order 'the usual'. I fear the closest I've ever come is sharing a bag of crisps and the latest on my love life with my favourite old fellas at the golf-club bar I once served behind. But, last week, I think I finally got the *Cheers*-like local of my dreams. Except the building is a hospital rather than a public house, the regulars are over-worked medical staff and my usual isn't so much a G&T as a strip to the waist and a flash of my boobs.

With P away on business, Tills came along instead, remarking how funny it was that I didn't have to check in at reception desks any more. And while treating hospital clinics like an office I've worked in for years could be seen as rather tragic, in fact it's a thing I enjoy. In I stroll, impossibly chirpy, offering a nod of acknowledgement to the fellow patients I've seen before and skipping the usual formalities with receptionists to talk trashy gossip instead of appointment times. Doctors usher me in with 'hi, Lisa' instead of 'Mrs Lynch please', greeting me in a manner that suggests we're about to catch up over a brew and biscuits, not discuss the scab on my left nipple.

'So nice to see you! I'm just looking at your breasts...' began Smiley Surgeon, in an opening line I'll never get used to (nor learn to stifle my sniggers upon hearing). '...and the symmetry is looking much better than last time. And wow, your nipple is healing really well,' he continued, promising to refer me to the nipple-tattooing nurse for an appointment in a couple of weeks' time. He's not wrong about the nupple – having now shrunk down to less grape-like levels, it's looking pretty damn good. So good, in fact, that I've been known on occasion to inflict on P a game of Spot The Falsie whenever my nipples are visible through a top.

Not everyone's so impressed with my new tit, mind you. Following a rather surreal conversation with Always-Right Breast Nurse about my post-treatment sex life and the best lubes on the market, she asked whether I'd be open to letting a recently diagnosed woman have a look at my surgery-sculpted bust. And since I'm so nonchalant about unbuttoning my shirt these days that I fear I'd remove my bra for the Sainsbury's delivery man if he asked nicely enough, I agreed. My nonchalance speaks volumes about how proud I am of the boob Smiley Surgeon has created for me. Having loved and lost a much-valued left'un, I never imagined I'd be so pleased with its replacement, and so I'm as keen to boast about my new baby as any first-time mother. But when I walked confidently into the next consulting room, I was as unprepared for the look on the poor woman's face as she was for the sight of my tit.

Was that the same terrified look I'd had in my eyes upon getting a similar world-changing diagnosis? I suspect so. She looked like she'd been hit by a train. Frightened, haunted, confused. Her tiny frame couldn't hold the weight of the worries she had to carry, just as her eyes couldn't hold back the tears she was trying to hide from her elderly mother. In her fifties and happily meandering through life until a week previous, she was due to undergo the same type of mastectomy with pre-reconstruction that I had (an LD-flap, fact-fans) and yet, with the gravity of the news she was still failing to compute, she couldn't get her head around what she'd find beneath her gown when she awoke from the op. And while my almost-finished result is, admittedly, quite different to the immediate post-surgery sight she'll be discovering any day now, Always-Right Breast Nurse figured that seeing Smiley Surgeon's second-to-none needlework would, in part at least, put her mind at rest.

But when I removed my vest and stood half-naked before her, she recoiled in horror. Literally. She took an instinctive step away from me, covering her mouth with her hands. Eventually, she leaned forward ever so slightly without moving her feet, her index finger covering her lips, as though she were inspecting a newly laid cat shit on her pristine carpet. 'Christ, woman. It's not that bad,' I thought, offended at her horrified reaction to my beautiful breast.

'I have to say, it doesn't look the same as your other one,' she said. Which was the moment at which I realised how far away from reality her expectations were.

'Well, no,' I replied, trying to remain as upbeat as I could. 'But you'd never be able to tell through my clothes. It's just that the new nipple looks pretty different to my old one. But even that's going to be tattooed.'

She inspected further, still a yard or two away. 'So – hang on – what happened to your old nipple?' she enquired.

'Um. It went,' I answered gingerly, looking over to Always-Right Breast Nurse in doubt about what to say next. She explained that the nipple has to be removed in order for the surgeon to work inside the breast, and that the replacement nipple she was looking at had been created with skin from my back.

'Coof,' she exhaled, correcting her posture and visibly shaking. 'There's just so much to take in.'

I grabbed her hand, telling her not to worry, then quickly realising what a pointless reassurance that was. 'Look,' I continued, 'you're right. There's more to take in right now than you can possibly get your head around, but soon, when you've had your surgery and your treatment has begun, I promise you'll feel a bit better because things will then be in hand. You'll be taking steps to make all this better. And it WILL get better,' I assured her, rather forcefully.

'Oh, the treatment,' she said, rolling her eyes. 'Did you lose your hair?'

For a second, I couldn't understand her question. 'Isn't it bloody obvious I've lost my hair?' I thought, then remembering that, in fact, I do have some hair now and that, to her, I was just a young lass with a short crop. I broke the news.

'I can't lose it,' she said. 'I just can't.' Hers was almost the same length that mine had been when I was in her shoes. 'Did you buy a wig?'

I nodded.

'And a headscarf?'

I nodded again, as she looked fit to puke. 'But, look, it's grown back,' I said, tugging at a few short strands. 'And I've had it cut and coloured since, too.'

She looked up and curiously inspected my head, with a defeated expression that said, 'But I don't want to look like that.'

'Nor do I, love,' I told her subliminally.

As I pulled my vest over my head, she went on to ask about the timescale of hair loss, how it felt to wear a wig and whether I kept my headscarf on in bed. Those odd little details that you must. know. now. despite the crash course in medical

265

terminology, despite the bigger issues at hand, despite the realisation that you've got a life-threatening condition. (I remember obsessing over the minutiae of how to draw on eyebrows, whether false eyelashes could look real, and how to ensure my husband never saw my bald head.)

'And chemo,' asked the woman, bringing up the subject I hoped she'd avoid. 'Were you very ill?'

I looked over at Always-Right Breast Nurse again, at a loss for what to say. How do you answer a question like that?

A-RBN chipped in: 'Chemo wasn't quite as bad as you'd expected it to be, was it, Lisa?'

Uncomfortable pause. I wanted to answer, 'No, it was a damn fucking sight worse,' but held back for the sake of the chemotherapy novice before me.

I was confused as to why Always-Right Breast Nurse had said that. Granted, I was hardly going to reel off the horrors of the hallucinations, the constipation, the bone aches or the looks on my parents' faces as I swore my way through barf after barf. But nor did I think it right to polish the turd that is chemotherapy. After all, I'd been sternly warned about how the treatment might affect my health and, while all the leaflets in the world couldn't have properly prepared me, at least I had some understanding that it was going to be pretty bloody shitty, thank you very much.

But then it dawned on me. For the first time I realised that, actually, I'd always made a point of playing down the effects of chemo to Smiley Surgeon and Always-Right Breast Nurse. I hadn't lied about it per se; I'd just never given them the full picture. And, having only ever seen them in my chemo 'good weeks', I could get away with it, too. Not just get away with it – I could pretend otherwise. So I'd tell them nothing more than that I'd had a turbulent couple of weeks, but that everything was fine now. No details. Just vagaries. I guess, too, that in those 'good weeks', I just didn't want to dredge it all up again. I was enjoying feeling more like a human being. Plus, of course, there's the suck-up in me who clearly put impressing my two favourite medical professionals before telling the not-so-impressive truth, wanting them to think I was some sort of super-patient for remaining so positive throughout something so utterly shitty; and batting away breast cancer as though it were dirt on my shoulder.

In the end, in fairness to the newly diagnosed woman in the consulting room, I plumped for a more enigmatic answer to Always-Right Breast Nurse's question. 'I'm not going to lie to you,' I half-lied. 'At times, chemo was a bitch. So I'm not sure about it being worse or better than I'd imagined. It was just very different to what I'd expected. But then the experience of chemo is utterly different for everybody.' I was still gripping her tiny hands. 'Of course it's not always easy. In fact, at times it's really bloody difficult. But, shit, it works. It did for me, and it will for you.'

She hugged me, as I grimaced nervously over her shoulder, hoping that I'd said the right thing. Always-Right Breast Nurse winked in my direction. Perhaps she knew the truthful answer anyway, despite my reluctance to give it.

*

'What do you mean you haven't got any summer clothes?' asked Kath over our lunch hour.

'Well, I threw them all away, didn't I?' I said. 'Which, with hindsight, might not have been my smartest decision.'

'Oh, and you were rocking such a good look before your diagnosis, too.'

'Meh,' I said, sipping my peppermint tea. 'I'm not exactly ready for a new summer wardrobe yet anyway.'

'What?' squealed Kath. 'You're going to Madrid! One of the fashion capitals of the world! You simply cannot be walking around in jeans and T-shirts, lady.'

'Well, I've got this,' I said tugging at the hem of my old faithful, take-me-anywhere black dress.

'And that's not going to do you,' warned Kath. 'It's all maxi dresses now, and cool shades and sassy handbags. Get yourself to Oxford Street, pronto.'

'But that's the end of our lunch hour!' I conceded. 'I'm flying tonight!'

'Then I'm ordering you to leave early today,' she insisted.

'Eh?'

'Consider it work. Your task for this afternoon is to get summer-ready.'

'If you say so, boss,' I relented, never one to stare into the gob of a gift horse.

'And while you're at it, sort yourself out with some Glasto clobber, too. Lisa Lynch, your summer of fun starts here.'

Kath wasn't the only one concerned with my summer-time preparation – there was another fairy godmother waiting for me *en España*. In her forties and before she met P's eldest brother Terry, my Spanish sister-in-law Paloma discovered that she had breast cancer. That diagnosis was more than eight years ago and today she's doing great. Better than great. She's a breezy, happy, no-messing, fun-seeking, beer-drinking, chain-smoking, newly retired heroine, and she was on brilliant form when we flew over to visit. 'You get the hot flushes, yes?' she said, thrusting a fan into my hand moments after we landed. She winked at me knowingly, smoothly opening her own fan and delicately waving it in front of her face in a single, seamless flick of the wrist. I returned the wink, trying to mimic her super-cool fanning manoeuvre but instead getting one of the prongs caught in my little finger and only extending it to what looked like a lacy, black slice of pizza. I was nervous; the clumsy Jedi Cancer Youngling to her Jedi Cancer Master.

It was a daft moment, really, but in that simple exchange of winks, I knew that she understood everything I'd felt over the past year; all the stuff I'd kept between me and Mr Marbles; all the feelings I'd not been able to explain to my family; all the things I'd not quite managed to describe on my blog. She just got it. No deep conversations, no tears, no confused Spanglish. Just a wink and a smile and a flick of a fan that said, 'Yep, I know.' (Or perhaps, 'The force is strong with you'. Whatever.)

The Spanglish route, however, was admittedly a more fun method of sharing our cancer stories, particularly since our respective Lynch boys have peskily ensured that the best we know of each other's languages is 'are you stupid or what?' (Paloma) and '*Cariño, he encogido a los niños*' (me).

'So, cheemoferathy,' she said, gallantly pronouncing the word better than I dare say I can in my mother tongue. 'Awful?' I raised my eyebrows in confirmation. 'Yep. Hell.' She agreed. 'Depression too, no?' We bobbed our heads like a pair of nodding dogs after three too many *cervezas*. 'And children? Is not possible?' (Insert obligatory nobody-expects-the-Spanish-inquisition gag here.) I shrugged, trotting out my now-standard line that P and I are happy enough, actually, and that life's just taken us down a different path, is all.

'Yes, we are lucky to have these men. I never really want to be a mother anyway,' said Paloma, as I caught our boys eavesdropping from the other side of the table, each with what looked suspiciously like an adoring glint in their eye. 'But you are okay,' she continued, in what I think was a statement rather than a question. 'When you arrive in the airport, I see your skin and I see your hair and I think, yes, you are fine; you are brave.' (See, the force is strong with me.) I gave her a cuddle, opting to swerve the mention of my hair and rest my usual routine of inflicting the hairdryer treatment on anyone who dared mention it.

As our conversation went on, though, it became eerily clear how similar our stories were, despite the almost-twenty-year gap in our ages at diagnosis. Left breast? Check. Stage three? Check. Oestrogen receptive? Check. No family history? Check. We talked of finding the lumps we each assumed were cysts; hers in the shower, mine in bed with P. I talked about Smiley Surgeon and his early advice to eat watercress and cherries. Paloma talked about her oncologist and his insistence that she should only eat red meat once in a while, drink a glass of red wine every day, have regular massages and to keep herself stress-free.

'Ah, that's my favourite piece of advice,' I said; though, oddly, it was my local shopkeeper rather than my oncologist who offered it to me. 'What you need to do, dear,' she insisted to me and Mum when I first made it the twenty yards to her store after Chemo 1, 'is remove all stress from your life. Work, money, worries, everything. Let everyone else take care of that. You just concentrate on you.'

It's fortunate that I was in a position to do that. My super-supportive company signed me off immediately, P took all the financial stuff in hand (not altogether a bad thing for a girl with an iTunes-and-handbag habit like mine), and my folks looked after the running of the flat whenever they were here. Everything just got done. The only stress I had was the one the tumour inflicted on me, which, frankly, was rather enough worry in the first place. Pre-cancer, however, my sister-in-law and I shared another similarity.

Around a year before we happened upon the evil activity beneath our left nipples, we both experienced a pretty rough ride in our jobs – the kind that finds you tetchy and sleep-deprived and makes you row with your husband for forcing you out of bed in the mornings.

'That kind of stress causes the cancer,' asserted my sister-in-law. I found myself half-heartedly agreeing out of politeness. She saw straight through me. 'No, no, it's true,' she assured me. 'My oncologist says it.' Now I'd only had a handful of sessions with my oncologist, but there was no way I could imagine Glamorous Assistant telling me that stress caused cancer any more than I could imagine her telling me to have a G&T every morning or that a diet of chocolate fondue would be a fast-track to better health. But Paloma's clearly believed it. As did she. And that's where our stories differed.

It's funny how a bit of sea can separate two countries' conclusions about The Bullshit. On this side of the Channel, it seems, we're far more careful about the semantics. Just as 'no trace of cancer' is acceptable where 'cancer free' isn't, I'm sure most British-based doctors would tap-dance around the statement that stress 'causes' cancer. And, from what I've gathered from my sister-in-law, Spanish oncologists place much more emphasis than their British counterparts on lifestyle and stress and attitude and positive thinking – those strange unquantifiables that can't be measured through a blood test. And though I didn't admit it in the course of that conversation, to my mind, that is a bloody risky strategy. We're supposed to be able to control stress, aren't we, lowering it as we would our cholesterol. So if stress leads to cancer, does that make those of us who've had it responsible? If we can't maintain a positive attitude, does that mean we're making things worse?

It's a funny one, this stress lark. Though I think there's only a very tenuous medical connection between stress and good health (in that some say it can weaken the immune system), I don't doubt that it plays a part. I have no basis to back it up but, at the risk of getting all new-age on you, I've always been a big believer in the link between the mental and the physical. Even at a simple level – blushing when you're embarrassed, shaking when you're nervous, working yourself up to the point of puke on the morning of your driving test, getting butterflies in your stomach before a first date. But suggesting that stress causes cancer? Sheesh. If that were the case, there'd be a chemo carriage on every underground train.

The problem, I think, is that it's human nature to search for answers. Why did this happen to me? Is it something I did wrong? What could I have done differently? So attributing stress to cancer might just be a case of finding an answer where there isn't one. And granted, in occasional moments of rage, I've blamed The Bullshit on my getting wound up by everything from shouty bosses to estate agents to bad referees to James Blunt. But in reality, I can't believe that. I can't believe it because that would make the cancer my fault. And there are plenty of things I'll take responsibility for – the pink nail varnish on our white bed linen, clogging up the Sky+ with episodes of *Hollyoaks*, having once had a crush on Mick Hucknall – but The Bullshit just ain't one of them. And tough as it is to come to terms with having nothing to blame it all on but a crappy combination of oestrogen and shit luck, that's just the way it's going to have to be. *Que sera sera.*

CHAPTER 34

Happy birthday

June 2009

'Oh, just be calm,' said the seen-it-all-before technician as I zipped up my dress after last week's yearly mammogram. 'Try to relax.' I turned green, bursting out of the seams of my frock.

'Relax?' I roared. 'RELAX?!' (I fear I became Brian Blessed for a moment.) 'How can I possibly relax? The last time I had one of these things,' I said, disdainfully pointing to the machine that had just squashed my right breast like a stress ball, 'it wasn't supposed to be a big deal, and I ended up with BREAST CANCER. I'm assuming it says that on your clipboard there?' I think she actually found my reaction funny, and sneaked out a little half-grin, demonstrably not believing that I was every bit as serious as the illness I'd been diagnosed with.

My last mammogram was done at Smiley Surgeon's clinic, mere minutes before my diagnosis. I hadn't even realised I'd be having one that day – as far as I was concerned, I was just going to the hospital to get the results of a 'routine biopsy' on my 'cyst'. And, given that I'd paid for that consultation in order to have it eight weeks sooner than I would have done on the NHS, it could all be done – the test, the results, the lot – in one day. By the time I'd re-dressed after my mammogram, the X-ray scans were already being printed out. And so, with this as my only melon-squeezing experience, I was optimistic that I'd know again this time – despite being in a different hospital – whether anything was awry on the day of my mammogram.

'I'll level with you,' I said to the technician as I unhooked my bra before she set the machine working. 'I'm really bloody frightened about this.' She half-grinned, in what was clearly her default unhelpful reaction to everything. 'And so I really want you to tell me if you see anything untoward,' I pleaded.

'I can't do that,' she snapped. 'I can't say anything; I'm not allowed. You have to wait to hear from the doctors.'

Tears fell from my eyes onto the edge of the machine before me. 'And how long is that going to be?' I whimpered.

'I'd say two to three weeks. They'll write to you. Or call. Sometimes they call.' I assumed 'sometimes' meant 'if there's a problem'.

I continued to cry as the machine did its thing, both from the pain of my flattened bust, and the pain of a protracted wait for my results. 'Okay, good,' said the technician as the whirring eventually ground to a halt. My head spun round in her direction. Was that 'good' as in there's nothing showing up, or good as in we're done? I daren't ask, for fear of the same I'm-not-telling-you reaction, and concern that my increasingly wounded-child-spliced-with-the-Incredible-Hulk demeanour would have seen me grab hold of her head and ram it between the same metal plates that had just turned my right tit to mincemeat.

And so now, we wait.

Again.

A-fucking-gain.

I'm holding it together as best I can, keeping as busy as my tiredness allows, and pretending I can ignore every sound from my phone or rattle of the letterbox. I'm trying to change any subject that relates to The Bullshit, push all negative thought to the back of my mind and work through all the anxiety-calming Q&A tactics Mr Marbles taught me to use whenever my worries find a way of surfacing. (Is this a rational thought? Do I have any reason to believe it's true? Can I back it up?) The trouble with that, though, is that my mind sometimes likes to play smartarse and think it's too clever for that kind of therapy malarkey. 'Well, yes, actually,' it'll say, sarcastically. 'That worry *is* rational and, yes, you do have reason to believe it and, yes, you can even back it up – hell, the last time you assumed your boobs were cancer-free, it came back to bite you on the ass good and proper, so screw Marbles and his calming tactics and keep tucking into those biscuits.'

But rational thought, of course, isn't necessarily about making yourself feel better. Ultimately, you've got to deal in fact. And so people can say 'you'll be okay' and 'there won't be a problem' and 'I just know it'll be fine' as much as they want, but do they really know that everything's going to be okay? Can they really feel it in their water? Of course not. No more than I can or the doctors can or The Piss-Taking God Of Cancer Fuck-Ups can. And so much of my focus at the moment is going into nodding politely whenever somebody does say something like that, and biting my lip to stop myself launching into a monologue about how I have to be open to receiving bad news, how I'm trying to prepare myself for the worst and how I'd hate to say I told you so if I got the kind of diagnosis that would satisfy nothing but my fondness for symmetry.

The shit truth here is that there's not a single sodding thing I can do about those unknown results either way. If there's cancer in my right boob (having had everything scooped out of the left, there was no reason to scan that side), then I'm just going to have to scream a few expletives, accept it, hitch up my skirt and wade through the swamp of whatever treatment they can give me for a second time.

And if there isn't any sign of further Bullshit then it's going to be one hell of a Glastonbury.

*

A year to the day that I was diagnosed with breast cancer, I was due to have my new nipple tattooed. I had been offered a couple of appointment slots that week, but figured that heading to the Nipple Clinic (how I wish it were really called that) on the day of my Bullshit anniversary was rather poetic and so, ever one to find the romance in a situation, I chose 17 June as the day on which I could replace the nipple that Smiley Surgeon suggested removing a year ago.

Even twelve months down the line I remained every bit as freaked out by my diagnosis as I was upon hearing it. *What, me? Breast cancer? Are you sure?* It still felt like I was talking about someone else – some poor sod I'd read about in a first-person magazine feature, or heard about in an eavesdropped conversation on the bus. It hadn't sunk in. It still hasn't sunk in. It may never sink in.

Having been for my mammogram a week previous, P and I had spent several days calling the hospital at least twice every twenty-four hours to check on the arrival of my results. The pair of us were as jumpy as kangaroos on a trampoline, and almost leapt out of our skins when a high-pitched voice called my name in the waiting room. I looked up to see who'd chirped so cheerily, and there stood a bubbly blonde burst of energy, all impressive eyeshadow and bright pink cardigan. Everything about her – her clothes, her make-up, her hair, her shoes – screamed 'colour is what I do'. The Pink Lady, as it turned out, was a breast care nurse by trade, but took additional training to become a nipple colour specialist who helps women replace the areolas that were lost as part of their mastectomies. I expect 'colour specialist' is the wrong title. It's bound to be something more medically impressive than that. Substitute Areola Consultant, perhaps, or Professor of Nipular Restoration.

At the beginning of my appointment, The Pink Lady passed me a photo album that filled my head with more images of boobs than a year's subscription to *Playboy*. As I flicked through the pages, I marvelled at 'before' pictures of one-nipple busts alongside 'after' photographs showing proud, completed racks of double-nippled glory. I tried to make all the right noises that suggested applause rather than arousal, but I dare say it was all a bit *Kinky Changing Rooms*, with tattooed areolas as *trompe l'œil* (Laurence Llewellyn Bowen would be proud), and with my tit as the next candidate for a makeover. And so The Pink Lady took out a Polaroid camera (I assumed she had to use an instant camera – I couldn't see the Boots processing counter turning a blind eye to a film full of tits) and took a photograph of my 'before' boob. During which, of course, I giggled like an idiot.

As I lay back on the bed, The Pink Lady leaned over me and inspected my non-nipple against my right one. 'Hmm,' she pondered. 'They're a lovely pale rose pink, aren't they?' I could have kissed her. What a wonderful compliment. It may have been the loveliest I'd ever had, and so I overlooked her use of the plural when I was demonstrably singular in the nipple department. 'I think we're going to need a very pale pink with a hint of fawn or brown,' she continued. As she buzzed away at my breast with exactly the same kind of tattoo-machine that had created the star on my wrist, I tried to think back to my days in interiors magazines, frantically attempting to recall the names of pink paints with a hint of fawn so I could freak her out with my own colour knowledge. 'Hm, yes, I imagine it's a good match for Farrow & Ball's Ointment Pink, wouldn't you say? Or Dulux Strawberries 'n' Cream, perhaps?' Thankfully, I stopped short of being such a smartarse, which is probably wise given my cheeks' tendency to turn Cinder Rose.

But, pleased as I was to have an optical illusion of a nupple whose colour almost resembled its mirror image, I couldn't help but be a teensy bit disappointed. With my new boob, the replacement silicone implant didn't just make up for the one that was taken away, but positively pissed on its bonfire with its perky, shapely, roundness. The replacement nipple, however, seemed to be merely the poor cousin to my right nipple. Because, as impressive as The Pink Lady's tattooing obviously is, it's not *that* good. And so I dare say that colouring in the twisted bit of skin that I call a nupple was a bit like putting Mac lipstick on a pig.

It might have been my attitude on that day, of course. Perhaps if I'd been for my nipple tattooing a week later, say, or even before my yearly mammogram, I'd have been in an altogether different frame of mind.

'How is it?' enquired P as I returned from the consultation room.

'It's, um, it's just meh,' I answered, unhelpfully.

'Meh?' repeated P.

'Meh. Just meh. You'll see,' I said.

'Okay, babe,' he said, carrying my handbag as we walked out of the clinic. 'So what now, then? Shall we head home and chill out?'

'Yeah, okay,' I agreed. 'But there's something I have to do first.'

Without needing clarification, P reached into my bag for the phone.

It wasn't just my desire for a happy cancerversary that led me to hope for news of a clear mammogram result on 17 June. For starters, I dreaded the thought of getting my results mid-Glastonbury, and learning half-cut in front of the Pyramid stage that my festival was being brought to an abrupt halt by yet more unwanted activity beneath my bra. By getting a clear result today, I thought, I could declare this Glastonbury *mine*, and enjoy it in the way I had intended since buying my tickets on that gloomy mid-chemo day in October. But bigger even than my hopes for a fun festival was my desire for a neat finish to this book. As I've revealed in the course of these pages, I'm a sucker for a clearly defined finish, and the thought of having to end this story on a cancer recurrence – or, worse still, an inconclusive result – worried me as much as the return of a tumour. I wanted this book to end tidily and exactly: A Year In The Life Of The Bullshit. I wanted to mark my first cancer anniversary like a particularly poignant birthday, and proudly declare the previous 365 days The Year I Wrote A Book – and not The Year I Had Cancer.

But, clear result or no clear result, even this foolish optimist knew that 17 June 2009 would not be the end of the road. There was plenty more to do. Because as much as the more hardcore phase of my Bullshit experience had tied itself up in a neat twelve months, the bigger battle was going to last a lifetime. And whether it was a year on from my diagnosis or thirty years on, I suspected the nervous, looming feeling I had in my belly as I called the hospital for my mammogram result would be exactly the same year upon year.

'Fuck, P, she's calling me back in a minute. That can't be good, can it?'

'What the? No. NO,' snapped P from the steering-wheel, his voice raising with every syllable. 'Tell me EXACTLY what she said.'

'She said she had my results in front of her but needed to talk to a doctor before she could tell me what they were.'

'Is that definitely what she told you?' bawled P accusatorily.

'Yes. Definitely . . . I think so. SHIT, P, I CAN'T THINK!'

'Why would she say that?' he screamed directly at the stream of tourists ignoring his right of way at Marble Arch. 'WHY THE FUCK WOULD SHE SAY THAT?'

'Ohgodohgodohgodohgod,' I mumbled, digging my nails into my thighs as I sat on my hands, rocking in the passenger seat.

When we got home, P and I tossed our bags into the living room and ourselves on the bed, lying back beside each other, staring up at the white ceiling in petrified silence. The phone rang.

'Sis! Fo shizzle ma nizzle,' sang Jamie from the other end of the receiver. 'What's goin' dow—'

'No-J-can't-now-waiting-for-mammogram-result,' I mumbled, turning my sentence into a single, unidentifiable word.

'Shit, okay. Laters,' he said, hanging up – turning from rapper to rapped in a nanosecond.

'Just Jamie,' I said to P, confirming what he already knew.

'Why does that always happen?' P whined. 'You can go a whole day without the sodding phone ringing and then just when you're expecting a big one . . .'

'Like buses,' I mumbled, too preoccupied to reply with anything other than the obvious cliché.

We resumed our position, side by side on the bed, with a couple of inches of white cotton separating us, too nervous even to allow our fingers to touch; inspecting the imperfections on a ceiling I'd come to know as well as the face in my mirror.

And then it came. 'This is it,' I said, recognising the caller ID. P sat upright and crossed his legs, holding his head in his hands in the same way he had after we'd discovered the severity of my diagnosis.

'Hi, this is Lisa, hi,' I answered, hurriedly. 'Can you tell me now?'

'Lisa, yes, sorry about that,' came the nurse's voice, pausing for a dramatic emphasis I didn't appreciate. 'It's clear.'

CHAPTER 35

Best foot forward

July 2009

During the Top 40 culmination of the tabloid-fest that was The Battle of Britpop, I was hanging by the scruff of my Fred Perry T-shirt off the railings at the back of my family's rented beach chalet, trying to get a radio signal to determine whether Blur or Oasis had come in at number one. I fear 'beach chalet' paints something of a misleading picture, actually – in truth it was a yellow, wasp-attracting wood-hut protecting the sleepy (nay, comatose) town of Sutton-on-Sea from the bitingly harsh (and, let's be honest, probably radioactive) Lincolnshire tide. It was where my family spent the same two weeks every summer and, in 1995, the soundtrack to my fortnight was Blur's 'Country House'.

Fast forward fourteen years to last Sunday night, somewhere halfway back in the crowd of Glastonbury's Pyramid stage and, as a newly reformed Blur played the same song, thoughts of wasp stings, chips with scraps and shaking sand out of my Adidas Sambas immediately filled my head. 'Country House' is by no means a terrific record, granted (and wasn't that just the irony of The Battle of Britpop?), but in a couple of bars' worth of oompah-ing brass, I was back in Sutton-on-Sea.

Given the link between pop songs and old memories, then, it's probably no coincidence that I've bought more albums in the last three months than I have in the entirety of the past year. You might consider that an odd decision, given that I've had so much time on my hands over the last twelve months that I could have easily reached recognising-songs-backwards familiarity with the combined back catalogues of everyone from Pink Floyd to Elvis Presley. But in truth, I didn't really pay much attention to music during my Bullshit year. It left an undisputed gap, I'll admit, but I put my indifference down to a simple lack of anything bordering on interest, energy or drive.

I wonder now, though, whether it might have been an unconscious decision not to muddy the soundtrack of 2008/09 with the worst time of my life? The one album I did embrace during that time (*The Seldom Seen Kid*, obvs), I made a point of only playing in times when I felt more like a human being, careful not to taint it with crappy cancer memories. I kind of hope my music-shunning was done on purpose, actually, because it might just be the smartest thing I ever did.

Getting to Glastonbury with P, Tills and Si (she says, as though it can be equated with reaching the summit of Everest or Nelson Mandela's *Long Walk To Freedom*) wasn't just a big deal in terms of how far I've come in the space of my 'gap year', but in recognising that it is possible to fall right back into the comforting arms of the stuff you love (or love listening to), like jumping off a perilous tightrope onto a huge, enveloping cushion. And the simple fact that it all happens on a farm in Somerset only adds to its brilliance. Because, when you're low on signal, when text messages are taking forty-eight hours to reach you and when you're miles away from your laptop and your email and your Twitter account, you're even further

283

removed from the communication-crammed life you couldn't do without back at home. And, strangely comforting as it is the rest of the time, you're not continually having to return hospital questionnaires or order repeat prescriptions or book follow-up appointments or answer questions several times a day about how you're feeling. And, by heck, it's glorious.

With a jolt, Si looked up from his pint of cider – or piss, we couldn't tell which – one afternoon at the festival. 'Crikey,' he said out of nowhere. 'I'd forgotten you'd even been ill.' And the beauty of it was – for the very first time in a year – I had too. Good old Glastonbury. You might come back bruised and muddy and covered in more germs than a Sunday-night portaloo, but any place that has the ability to make you forget about The Bullshit gets a McCartney-style thumbs-up from me. And so those four days on Worthy Farm marked more than just a brilliant Blur reunion, the return to fashion of Springsteen-like sweatbands and the realisation that Neil Young can make 'Down By The River' last for three weeks. It also marked the moment when I took my finger off the pause button and finally pressed play on my lovely life once more.

*

'If someone could have told me a year ago,' said P, as we kept each other warm in front of a candle flame on our old-person blanket at rock 'n' roll's biggest festival, 'that we'd be here and you'd be better, well . . .'

'Well?' I queried.

'Well, y'know, I s'pose I'd settle for that,' he concluded, in what could almost certainly take the gong for the World's Largest Understatement.

'Yeah, I probably would too,' I agreed, mimicking his dryness.

Months previous, some smart cookie had commented on my blog that one day I'd turn around to notice that things had become normal again, without even realising they had got that way. And in that cidered-up conversation in the cold, in which cancer was just a mere detail for my husband and I to trivialise, I guess it finally happened.

For over a year, I had been longing to have a chat that didn't begin with my diagnosis or my hair or the state of my immune system or my scars or my infection or my hot flushes or my boobs. I'd lost count of the number of people who'd opened telephone calls with 'how are you feeling?' instead of 'hello'. It was overwhelmingly lovely that every-one had so much invested in me getting better, and that they were so interested in what stage I was at with my recovery. But the repeated questions about my well-being also meant that something must have been wrong.

And so, even more than I was searching for a cancer cure or a tumour-free boob or a good head of hair or a new nipple, I was searching for normality. The kind of normality in which I could talk *Coronation Street* before cancer. In which I'd be sick because I'd had too much to drink, and not because of chemo. Where people would ask 'how's things?' instead of 'how are you feeling today?' The kind of normality in which I could moan about my hair despite once not having had any, or whinge about the size of my thighs as though their enormity were the worst thing that could possibly happen to me. In which our families could visit for a weekend because they wanted to say hi, and not because they had to look after us. And in which I could tell my husband I loved him because I felt like it, and not because I was worried how many more times I might be able to say it. The kind of normality in which I could sit on a blanket in a field, rather than under a blanket on my sofa.

The kind of normality in which I could be just another face in an 180,000-strong crowd.

And so, yeah, I'd seen off treatment for breast cancer. But I didn't necessarily want to be hailed a hero for doing it. I just wanted to be an ordinary girl, living an ordinary life – just as I had been before The Bullshit. I wanted to be able to answer my dad's daily question of 'what's your news?' with a boring 'bugger all', and for him to respond with a satisfied 'that'll do for me'. And while it would be far too worthy – and a complete fabrication – of me to tell you that there wasn't a significant part of me that wanted to stop every Glasto punter in their tracks and say 'guess what – I survived breast cancer' in the hope of them buying me a congratulatory beer, I also knew that surviving The Bullshit wasn't necessarily something I could take the credit for. Because I didn't beat cancer. I just had the kind of cancer that could be treated, and a brilliant medical team to see to its eradication. My job was simply to allow them to do it; to accept the treatment; to accept the way that treatment would make me look and feel, and to hope for the best.

But since all that's a bit zen, and since I'm also the kind of girl who (a) prefers a burn-out to a fade-away, and (b) will never pass up the opportunity to claim a reward, I roped P into a rather special, post-Glastonbury shopping trip.

'I'm getting these,' he said.

'No, *I* am,' I protested, wondering why we were arguing about who'd hand over the card from our joint account.

'But *I* want to do the buying,' bickered P.

'Fine,' I conceded. 'But if anyone asks, for the record, I bought them for myself. As a present to *myself*. Right?'

'Yeah, whatever,' he said, raising a suspicious eyebrow at the goods in the shop window.

If you ignore the fact that we had to ring a doorbell to get into the shop, and that I had a dedicated and impossibly helpful assistant, this was as normal a Saturday-afternoon shopping experience as P and I had ever had: me spending far longer than is necessary making confused faces in front of a mirror; him standing awkwardly in a corner checking the cricket score on his phone.

'Peeeee,' I whined. 'Give me an honest opinion! This one or this one?'

'Um, walk over there,' he said, putting his phone behind his back but clearly keeping one finger on a button so as not to lose his page. 'Dunno babe. *You've* got to wear them.'

'And *you've* got to look at them,' I retorted.

'Dunno. Like 'em both,' he concluded.

'Well, that's helpful,' I said, turning to the assistant in invitation for some audience participation in the man-and-wife shopping routine we'd been honing for years. 'The thing is,' I told her as P got back to a fallen wicket, 'I want to wear these *for ever*. If I'm going to spend this much money, they've got to go with *everything*.' I figured it would be fruitless to pretend that we went on these kind of sprees all the time, utterly obvious as it was that we were more used to shopping in Kennington than Knightsbridge.

'In which case I think you're along the right lines with either of these,' she answered politely, backing up the opinion that P had almost given.

I gurned a bit more in front of the mirror before turning to P. 'These,' I said, pointing to my right foot. 'It's these.'

'And you're sure?' asked P, as he exchanged his credit card for an expensive-looking brown carrier bag. 'It's a big deal, is this.'

'Damn right it's a big deal,' I agreed.

*

'I'm just going to watch these last couple of overs while you play with your new toy,' said P, stretching out on the sofa after coping admirably with a couple of hours of enforced girliness. With the fragments of our festival still scattered around the bedroom, I made some space on the bed amidst our rucksacks and rain macs to release my Best Ever Purchase from its box. Shooing dirty clothes underneath the bed to clear the floor between me and the mirror, I kicked aside my muddy wellies and took the first tentative steps in my peep-toe Christian Louboutins.

'Haha!' I squealed excitedly at my 6 foot 1 reflection, throwing my arms out and barely staying upright in an emancipated wobble. In the aftermath of breast cancer, I was already having to learn to walk again – and here I was adding 12-centimetre heels to the equation. But after a Bullshit year of extraordinary trials in which I could only *hope* to stand this tall, I figured this ordinary girl was ready for a new challenge.

Acknowledgements

With thanks . . .

I've spent my life reading bands' acknowledgements in album sleeves and have always dreamt of one day doing the same, so please forgive me for lapping this up like a hungry sales shopper on New Year's Day.

I'd like to thank ~~the Academy~~ the following people, not just for the part they played in getting this book to print, but for the part they played in dragging me through the bullshit that was The Bullshit.

Firstly, to all the amazing internet friends (ooh, friend) who've ever read, linked to, commented on, RTd, passed around or pimped out *Alright Tit*. I kiss you all on both cheeks. To Marsha Shandur, who got in there early, always one step ahead of the game. To Stan Cattermole, for the post that sent his discerning readers my way. To Stuart Bradbury, for the brilliant blog design that got me noticed. To Matt Thomas, for nagging me to join Twitter. To Stephen Fry, for driving my traffic sky-high with his kind words.

To Kath, for being the best (and brilliantly bad-influence) boss, and everyone else at Forward. To Shirley, for regular thoughtful emails and enough flowers to start a pot pourri-business. To Mr Bancroft, who I always said I'd thank if ever I wrote a book. To Dave Grohl, for ignoring the constant stalker-like references. (My final thinly veiled attempt at getting him to notice me.) To Derby County, for staying up in a season when I couldn't have handled relegation. To Sgt Pepper, for forcing me into breaks by sitting on my keyboard (any typos are her fault, by the way), and for changing me more than cancer ever could.

To my agent Matthew Hamilton, for discovering my writing and always sharing good news in time for the weekend. To everyone at Arrow, in particular Steph Sweeney, Gillian Holmes, Claire Round, Louisa Gibbs, Charlotte Bush, Amelia Harvell, Richard Ogle, David Wardle and the sales team for their staggering enthusiasm and belief in *The C-Word*, and the hard work (and hard drinking) that got it to print.

To every single medical professional at the London Breast Institute and Royal Marsden Hospital (the most remarkable of whom are mentioned in this book) whose expertise helped get me to this point. I owe you everything. But for now, this acknowledgement and a few fairy cakes will have to do.

To all of my wonderfully supportive friends who have, from my very first blog post, been relentlessly encouraging to pushy-showbiz-mother levels. In particular, the darling Tills, for always finding something nice to do in Chemo Week 3 and stepping up to be the sister I never had; and Si, for on-tap DIY assistance and funny-shaped crisps. To Ant, for staying unreservedly local despite being so far away. To Polly and Martin, for the most gloriously relieved reactions when my mammogram was clear. And to our 'Goldsmiths Mum' Angela, for taking off the caps lock. To Weeza, for making my life better by simply being back in it. To Busby, for the comedy ginger wig and planting the Super Sweet seed. To Lil, for always ensuring that normal conversation prevailed, and for being Sgt Pepper's favourite auntie; and Sal and Ive, for *Abigail's Party* and colour-coordinated get-well cards. To Ali, for endless cheery cups of tea; and Leaks, for *never* taking it seriously. To The WardJonze Entity, for twelve years of toilet humour and the book we've not yet written. To Jon, Suze and the boys, for making P and I part of your lovely family. And to every other impossible-to-list mate who's ever called, cuddled, poked, emailed, visited, texted, baked me gingerbread men or bought me a curly scouse wig. Even the ones who just didn't know what to say.

To the Lynch clan – Val, Terry, Ted, Paloma, Andy, Tracey, Izzy, John, Val (and the extended scouse relatives it'd take me another book to list) – a family force to be reckoned with. Let's celebrate in The Star soon, eh?

To Jean and Hedley, for always making me feel like I was on the right track. To Paul, for donating an obscene amount to Breast Cancer Care for the first copy of this book. To Will, for Googling breast cancer when he should have been knee-deep in Lego. To Non, for staying characteristically calm. To Auntie Anne, my cancer buddy, heroine and Matriarch To End All Matriarchs. To Uncle Frank, for the most wonderful cuddles. To Matthew, for Isle of Wight escapes and scrambled eggs with leftover curry. And to everyone else I'm fortunate enough to call family or family-friend.

To Jamie, the most thoughtful, kindest, loving, funniest, arse-faced, piss-taking brother there ever was. And to his beautiful Leanne, for being brave enough to marry into the Macs (and well worthy of the name). To my incredible Mum and Dad, for EVERYTHING. Even in the darkest hours of

The Bullshit, I never felt anything less than bloody lucky to have been born to such an exceptional couple. I hope you know what an extraordinarily envied family you've created.

And – finally and most importantly – to my pride and joy, my reason, my world, my everything: my P.

What Happened Next

The C Word ends in June 2009, but Lisa continued to write her blog. So if you'd like to read more of Lisa's story, here are a few of her warm and witty posts written after *The C Word* was published. They cover everything from her never-ending love for Dave Grohl (of course), to the brilliance of Trinity Hospice.

If you'd like to make a donation to Trinity Hospice, their website is http://www.trinityhospice.org.uk

Geek like me.

'I have NEVER seen you like that,' huffed P as we pulled away from the hospital following our last appointment with Smiley Surgeon.

'You haaaave,' I chirped confidently. (A rather misplaced confidence, given the masterclass in goondom I'd just performed in my surgeon's office.)

'Why do you go all high-pitched?' he quizzed, now mimicking my tone. 'You're all *"Hi! I'm Lisa Lynch! I'm friendly and cheerful! Please love me!"* And all in that weird voice you do.'

'Fuck off,' I spat, in an altogether lower octave.

'Seriously though, babe, you're a proper goof.'

'I can't help it!' I squealed. 'Honestly! I sit in that waiting room giving myself little pep-talks before every appointment. "Don't do it this time, Lis. Play it cool, Lis. Act normal, Lis." But when I get in there it all turns to shit. I literally have no control over it. It's chemical.'

P continued to skit me. 'And all that stuff about The Curly Professor. *"Ooh, and he told me to pass on his regards, and to tell you that you've done a really excellent job!"* I mean, come on, woman.'

'But he *did* say that!' I protested.

'I know he did. But it's the *way* you say it. You're such a massive fucking suck-up.'

'Oh, just... sod off,' I sulked, as P near pissed himself laughing.

At the risk of making excuses for myself when I ought to be waving a giant white flag, I do think that there was a bloody good reason for my added goondom this time. A couple of bloody good reasons, in fact.

For one, Smiley Surgeon didn't just agree with The Curly Professor's prophylactic-mastectomy-and-oophorectomy advice, but went one – nay, two – better by suggesting that they could both be done this autumn (*this autumn!*) and – crucially – at the same time (*the same time!*). And after hearing that, of course, I damn near crawled across his desk and hugged the glasses clean off his face.

My second goon-excuse, though, is that this was the appointment during which I was to give Smiley Surgeon – as I'd promised the last time I saw him – an early copy of my book. (Which, by the way, is out in two weeks and available to pre-order from all good online retailers. *double thumbs up*) And so, despite the gravity of the stuff we were talking about in our consultation, the high-pitched voice in my head persisted in reminding me about the gift I had to give him all the way through our session.

'*You mustn't forget the book!*' the voice chided as Smiley Surgeon examined my bothersome boobs.

'*But don't make a massive deal of it!*' it pestered as he declared that he'd be able to preserve my right nipple. (*Preserve my nipple!* Actually, make that goon-excuse #3.)

'*And don't mention that he's in it!*' it nagged as he made me

296

aware of the small yet positive impact that preventative surgery could have on my life expectancy.

'Just slide it across the desk and be outta here!' it teased as he promised to refer me to a gynaecological surgeon to discuss the details of my oophorectomy.

And then it was my turn.

'So does that answer all your questions?' Smiley Surgeon asked after talking me through everything I needed to know.

'I think so, yep,' I said, doing what I could to talk above my inner voice. 'So I guess I'll have my MRI done and then come back to you for the mammogram in June, and then if all the scans are clear I s'pose we can crack on.' (I actually said 'crack on'. Like we were talking about a haircut, and not the removal of my ladybits.)

'Indeed,' he said.

'Cool,' I said.

'So if that's it, then…' Smiley Surgeon concluded, pushing himself up from the arms of his chair.

'Actually, um… there is one more thing,' I stuttered, getting squeakier with every syllable. 'Remember how I told you about my book?'

'Oh yes! Have you got it?' he asked, enthusiastically.

'Well, this is your copy,' I said, sliding it across the desk as the voice had advised.

'Brilliant!' he exclaimed, turning it over to look at the back cover. 'Brilliant! And a quote from *The Telegraph*! That's very prestigious!'

'Oh heck, don't get your hopes up,' I goofed, as he continued to read the blurb.

It was at this point that I suddenly remembered the horribly soppy message I'd written inside the cover. Fuck – the message! *'An acknowledgement in a book doesn't quite cut it…'* Oh fuckshitbollocks. *'Thank you for giving me a breast I've come to love every bit as much as the one I lost…'* And, oh no – double fuckshitbollocks – the massive kiss! And the heart! In pink pen! What the fuck had I done? I'll tell you what I'd done. I'd just handed the man responsible for my cancer-prevention a book in which I swear like a trooper, talk at length about my bowel movements, and reveal that I'm a little bit in love with the doctors who've treated me. A book in which he doesn't even know he's a major character. A major character with a pet name, ferfuckssake.

'Abort mission! Abort mission!' screamed the voice in my head. *'Pick up your bag! Leave the building! Get the fuck out! NOW!'* Panicked adrenaline forced me out of my seat and into my jacket in a single flinch.

Smiley Surgeon continued to hold up my book's cover at his eye level, and proudly turned it around to show the trainee surgeon who'd been observing our appointment. I'd barely even noticed she was there.

'This is amazing, Lisa,' he said, taking his smiley moniker to new levels.

I shrugged and blushed simultaneously, as P made a gesture that suggested we ought to be leaving.

'It's great that you've turned all of this into something so positive,' Smiley Surgeon went on. Which, of course, made me blush even more.

'Pahh,' I burbled, maniacally waving a hand in front of my face in the hope of passing off my reddening cheeks as a hot flush.

'My, you are determined,' he said, bringing our meeting to a close as I sheepishly skulked out of the room.

'Yup,' said the voice in my head. 'You're determined, all right. Determined to make yourself look like the right tit he's going to remove.'

'Scuse me while I kiss the sky.

MONDAY, 6 SEPTEMBER 2010

I recently said to my mate Weeza that it's a wonder my post-Bullshit life hasn't turned me to drink, given how often it makes me feel like a manic depressive. I've talked before about the high highs and low lows that are my life; and how the days of blissful boringness are so few and far between that my existence is less of a rollercoaster than an eternally bouncing bungee cord, alternating wildly between free-falls into the grand canyon and head-rushing catapults towards the space station. Bouts of chemo tempered with kind tweets from Stephen Fry; scan-result anxiety set against book-launch excitement; apprehension about next week's surgery juxtaposed with letters from Dave Grohl…

Oh, I'm sorry – did I just say 'letters from Dave Grohl'? Oh dear. Did I let it slip that Dave 'top of my list' Grohl has *written me a letter*? And did I also mention that he's signed a copy of my book?

Did I? Did I actually say that stuff out loud? Hm? Did I?

Too fucking right I did.

'I've got an amazing birthday present for you,' said my LA-based mate Ant. 'You can't have it for a while yet but I can't wait any longer to tell you about it.'

'Ooh! What?'

'Well, remember I told you that my brother's ex knew someone who worked as Dave Grohl's assistant...?'

I obliged her drumroll of a hint with a couple of seconds of dramatic-effect silence.

'Well, she's got something for you. ... A letter. ... From *Grohl himself*.'

'You're fucking kidding me!' I yelped in startling high-pitch, sending every dog in south London into an epileptic fit. 'Squeeeeeeeeeeeeeee!'

'And he's signed a copy of your book as well.'

'Fuck off! Fuck right off! You're joking! MY book? He's ACTUALLY HELD a copy of MY BOOK?'

'Yup.'

'He held it in his hands? In his ACTUAL HANDS?'

'Oh, um, you've gone all weird.'

'Sorreee! But omigodomigodomigod it's just *ah-may-zi*... Peeeeeeeeee!' I interrupted myself, squealing through the flat, 'Ant's got me a letter from Dave Grohl! An ACTUAL letter! And he's signed a copy of my book! My ACTUAL book! Signed by Dave Grohl! Eeeeeeeee!'

'That's great, love,' came the unruffled response from the kitchen.

'Eeeep! What does it say?' I squeaked into the receiver. 'Whatdoesitsay? Whatdoesitsay? Doyouknowwhatitsays?'

'No, I've no idea,' said Ant, sidestepping the urge to suggest that it's probably less marriage-proposal than cease-and-desist order. 'But it's going to get dropped off with me in LA and then I'll post it onto you, so it might be a couple of months til you get it.'

'Oh, bird – that *genuinely* doesn't matter. Omigodomigodomigod. An ACTUAL letter. And I *know* it's coming. Mate, I can wait FOREVER. Omigodomigodomigod.'

'Er, Mac… you've gone all strange again.'

On this occasion, then, you might forgive the following fate-tempting words when I say that, lately, it feels a little like the balance of my maniacal moods has tipped, and that the tide is getting promisingly higher on my luck-levels.

Well, I say 'lately'. That's a bit of a fib, actually, given that I've been sitting on my next bit of good fortune for a wee while, but it's only now that I am able to unzip my gob and finally – *officially* – spill the goods. (A bit like my wonderfully over-excitable brother who spends every November badgering you to let him reveal what he's got you for Christmas, only to drop a massive clanger of an it-plays-DVDs style hint at 11pm on Christmas Eve.) So, if you thought I'd lost my ability to play it cool – ha, as if it ever existed – with The Dave Grohl News, then try this on for size: the BBC are developing an adaptation of *The C-Word*.

*happydances on spot, screams like the kid in *Little Miss Sunshine*, checks pulse to confirm hasn't died and gone to heaven*

Yup, an adaptation! Of my book! An ACTUAL dramatic adaptation! For 90 ACTUAL minutes! In development by the ACTUAL BBC, courtesy of the ACTUAL executive-producing genius that is the ACTUAL Susan Hogg! For the ACTUAL telly! On the ACTUAL BBC1! Played by ACTUAL actors! With an ACTUAL… okay, you get it. See what I mean about cracking my head against the space station?

So yeah, welcome to my increasingly surreal life. This week, for instance, has been a brilliantly bipolar blend of worrying myself into borderline catatonia about next week's surgery and – cue hypomania – grinning myself into excitement-induced insomnia thinking about who might play me. (And P. And Jamie. And Mum. And Dad. And Tills. And Smiley Surgeon. And Sgt Pepper.) One minute it's depression, the next it's delirium; my only mood-stabilizer being the bafflingly accidental development of my ability to fall into a skip-full of shit and somehow clamber out smelling like a Jo Malone flagship store.

My mates are endlessly entertained by all this, of course, but what none of them can agree on is whether you'd call my crazy fortunes inherently good or bad? 'If we didn't love you so much,' said one friend after my back-break, 'I think we'd all probably think twice about being mates with such an unlucky person.' 'I mean, publishing a book!' said another after *The C-Word*'s release. 'You're such a lucky bitch! I'd love for that to happen to me.'

But which friend was right? Let's look at the evidence. Girl born to wonderful family, has happy life, meets fantastic boy, gets married, has miscarriages, discovers cancer, loses left tit, writes blog, loses hair, gets better, enters menopause, discovers BRCA gene, publishes book, breaks back, loses right tit and ovaries, gets letter from Dave Grohl, has film made about life… I mean, Jaysus, I sure as heck don't know which way to call it. (No bloody wonder this is being developed into a drama.)

So – lucky bitch? Unlucky bitch? There's probably a bit of truth in both, and thus I don't mind either way… people can come to whatever conclusion they like. But, as I'm sure anyone would agree, one thing you can *never* say is that this – whether intentional or otherwise – is anything other than the very definition of milking The Bullshit for all its worth.

What was it a wise man once said? Oh aye – when life gives you lemons, grab the tequila.

A matter of time.

8 June 2012

Ordinarily, when I've been away from social media for a while, it's a sign that all is not well. As any of my mates will tell you, I have a somewhat useless habit of 'going under' for a few days (all right, *weeks*) when things are particularly shitty, generally waiting until someone forces the problem out of me before I do anything about it. This last month or so, however, has been rather different. My lack of Twittering or Facebooking or whatever isn't the result of a turbulent period, but instead the result of that most glorious of time-fillers: normality.

It's all thanks to my treatment break, of course: a timely, precious and enormously appreciated stretch in which my social activity is – *finally* – more actual than virtual. I've spent time back home with the family, been out for swanky dinners, seen more of my mates, had weekend escapes in lovely hotels, spent a gorgeous week in Spain (so gorgeous, in fact, that we're off there again tomorrow), been to gigs, attended a lovely wedding, had my friend Ant from LA over to stay, thrown a Jubilee party... in short, I've squeezed in the all the life I wasn't able to live while on seven months' worth of chemo into seven weeks' worth of chemo-break. It's been bloody wonderful. And, given that this well-earned rest is teetering on a could-end-at-any-moment precipice, I'm buggered if I'm calling a halt to the fun just yet. Life, I've come to learn, is very simply about making time for happy memories and spending time with the people you love – and that's what I'll continue to do, until such a time as The Bullshit creeps back to piss on my chips, when I'll scrap with all I've got to get back to this; the good stuff.

The only problem with such a situation, however, is that there are more demands on my time than perhaps ever before. And in these days of uninhibited openness, constant narration, candid diarising and ever-growing friendship circles – particularly through the likes of blogging and social media – it can prove tricky terrain to negotiate, and I'm conscious of coming across as the kind of person who uses those tools only in times of dire need, ditching them (and anyone associated with them) when things are looking up. The truth of the matter, though, is that – as an advocate of the sharing culture that social media has granted us – I want to let everyone in on the good as well as the bad. It's just, I suppose, that when things are better, and you're so desperate to drink it up, it leaves less space to do so, and hence just *living* takes precedence over *sharing* that living. And, you might say, quite rightly too.

Since we're talking truths, though, there's even more to it than that. Because, see, in this wonderful period of living, it's not just my lack of *time* to share my narrative that's making me look somewhat on the quiet side, but my lack of inclination. Since September last year, all I've had to think about is how I'm feeling, how long I've got, and whether my treatment is worth the trauma. But now, all of a sudden, those things – permanently etched into my mind though they remain – have been allowed to sit on the back-burner, gifting me time to think about the more important things in life, like what to buy people for their birthday, whether my nails match my outfit, and what to delete on the Sky+ to make way for more *Jersey Shore*...all of which have, on a number of occasions, taken precedence over blogging or tweeting or replying to Facebook messages or emails. In short, I suppose, where previously my brain's been filled with Bullshit, now it's filled with bullshit. And so it's no surprise that where the cancer crap is concerned, lately, I just don't want to talk about it.

I apologise if that's a confusing message to send out, particularly when we all know that there'll shortly come a time when I'll *have* to (heck, *want* to) talk about it once more. Right now, though, I'm just so over it that I'm, I dunno, under it. Which, granted, is a bit on the ridiculous side when you're supposed to be keeping up a blog on the progress of your health.

Another confusing message I may have sent out – okay, *overused* – is the one that goes thus: 'Yeah, definitely! As soon as I'm on my treatment break...' Talk about stitching yourself up, eh? Because, with the disproportionate amount of time spent in treatment than out of it, there's only so many times you can come good on that promise – particularly when it comes to the friends I've never met; the folk whose virtual kindness has been so helpful to me through years of The Bullshit.

The odd person has become impatient with me – angry, even – as a result of this state of affairs, but what those virtual friends perhaps don't know – where my real-life friends do – is how much of a knock my confidence has taken over the last few months. Where once I was poised and self-assured and perfectly fine when it came to meeting new people, now I only feel confident in the company of my very closest family and friends. Thus, when you add that side-effect to the lack of time in which I have to see my nearest and dearest before everything goes tits up again, the result is a lovely big dollop of guilt about how my treatment break — my timely, precious, enormously appreciated treatment break — is spent.

In many ways it's classic me, this, isn't it: finding stuff to fret about in the very period I ought to be fret-free, but old dogs and new tricks n' all that. You might call it fatalistic; but I call it funny (albeit the sick side of funny). Because, hey — in the grand scheme of worries, these are pretty bloody lovely worries to have. And let me tell you, it ain't half nice to know that, even after a months-to-live talk, you're capable of going back to fretting about daft stuff like how much time you spend updating your Twitter feed.

So I do hope you'll excuse me if I smirk my way back to Spain this weekend. But please don't be offended if you don't get a postcard, eh? Chances are I'll just be having too much fun to write one.

A birthday wish.

6 August 2012

Dear family and friends,

Later this month it's my birthday. I'll be 33, like a long-playing record, or the temperate at which water boils. Or, interestingly (/uninterestingly), the one age I'm likely to share with Sgt Pepper. (In cat years, like. I'm not 4. Just to clarify.)

Anyway, yes, birthday. There was only one thing I wanted for my birthday: to make it there. And, provided I can avoid getting sawn in half, tripping over boxes marked 'TNT', and keep away from falling pianos on the run-up to the 30th, I think we can safely say I've done it. So what else do I want for my birthday? (Aah, 33 years of 'I want doesn't get' utterly wasted eh, Mum and Dad?)

Well, since you ask, there *is* something I'd like, please. (Pah, as if my parents didn't drill politeness into me from the womb.) Just one thing. And it's pretty simple. See, with my birthday in mind, I've been looking at my life in terms of the things that I need. Not the working-iPhone, Mulberry-handbag, three-pairs-of-Converse stuff, because ~~I'm a jammy bugger who's already got that covered~~ that doesn't matter, in the grand scheme of it all. And so, what I realised I really *do* need, then, is to continue my life in the manner in which it's currently being lived: sometimes expectantly, sometimes anxiously – but, ultimately, happily.

But where the hell can you find the wrapping paper for that, eh? Well, that's kind of the point: I don't want you to buy wrapping paper. Or, for that matter, a card. And more to the point, I don't want (sorry – *wouldn't like*) you to buy me a present, either. Because, as suggested in the above paragraph, there's something I need a lot more instead.

As no doubt you've heard from me over the last few months, I've been spending some time – every Thursday, actually – at Trinity Hospice. (Yeah, I shuddered the first time I heard that, too. Turns out, though, it could easily rival Disneyland for that 'happiest place on earth' title. And if you don't believe me, come along one Thursday and I'll be happy to prove you wrong.)

It took a rather unadvised handful of anti-anxiety pills to even get me out the door on my first visit, so shot to shit was my confidence. But, as I later explained <u>in this blog post</u>, Trinity's mobility-bus driver Mick, who came to pick me up, assured me that the happy-go-lucky girl I once was would be coaxed out again, with the help of the day staff at Trinity's day centre, Mulberry Place.

Thursdays have since become the jewel in the crown of my week. I've benefited from physiotherapy, worked my way through some tough-ass psychotherapy (and some much gentler counselling), learned new skills and made new friends. And, granted, those friends are more than a few ~~generations~~years older than me, but they're mates in the truest sense of the word: we love each other's company, we can talk about *anything* (and equally, nothing), we constantly take the piss out of one another, gossip like teenagers on a lunch break, we've got each other's backs, and have each contributed towards the building of an enormously special dynamic. Seriously, if we weren't all so bloody sick, we'd be the Avengers or something.

The aim of the staff at Mulberry Place is to "improve wellbeing by building the confidence of patients, families and carers; helping them to find ways to cope with what may be an uncertain and challenging future." All of this care – both at Mulberry Place and Trinity's in-patient wing – is provided free of charge, yet only one third of its funding comes from the government. Without the £6 million raised in charity every year, Trinity Hospice simply wouldn't exist. (And £6 million is a heckofa lot to ask for a local charity.)

Which brings me back to my birthday, and my wishes for it. I'm lucky enough to have an incomparable husband, an exceptional family and truly wonderful friends. I have a lovely flat, with a wonderful cat and a fully-stocked fridge. I have the ability to work, enough money in the bank to keep me in Tunnock's Teacakes (or, more to the point, mini Twister lollies – The New Tunnock's^{TM}) and, for now at least, I have my health. But despite the combined brilliance of everything and every person above, when I found myself in a sickeningly depressing, post-treatment slump of terrifying uncertainty, only one thing was able to bring me back to life: Mulberry Place, and all the superbly rehabilitative, healing, restorative magic that goes on within its doors.

Thus when I said that what I'd like for my birthday is to continue my life in the manner in which it's currently being lived, I'm sure you can appreciate how integral Trinity Hospice is to that. So, please: no presents or cards this year (I won't be in the country to accept them anyway) – how about visiting the below web page and giving whatever you might've spent to Trinity Hospice instead? (Or, more specifically, to Mulberry Place, which is where I have asked that any money raised on this page be apportioned.)

There is, quite genuinely, nothing else I need... nothing except my Thursdays, and all the lovely things I already have in my life. So let's save the festivity-type-stuff for another time, yeah? Maybe for when I make it to 34. Because hey, who wouldn't want to celebrate being the same age as the atomic number of selenium, or the dialling-code for Spain, eh? Oh aye. 34. We'll go mad then.

With all my love,
Happy-go-lucky Lisa x

PS: Obviously, not all of you reading this are in the circle obliged to know my birth date – and thus, of course, I absolutely don't expect you to contribute towards my birthday fund for Mulberry Place. What you might like to do instead, however, is help me spread the word about how wonderful Trinity are, whether by <u>sharing this post</u>, learning a little more about the hospice <u>via their website - http://www.trinityhospice.org.uk/</u>, or even by offering your services as a volunteer.